AF587891

Neurology – Laboratory and Clinical Research Developments Series

INTRACRANIAL HYPERTENSION

NEUROLOGY – LABORATORY AND CLINICAL RESEARCH DEVELOPMENTS SERIES

Intracranial Hypertension
Stefan Mircea Iencean and Alexandru Vladimir Ciurea
2009 ISBN: 978-1-60741-862-7

Neurology – Laboratory and Clinical Research Developments Series

INTRACRANIAL HYPERTENSION

STEFAN MIRCEA IENCEAN
AND
ALEXANDRU VLADIMIR CIUREA

Nova Biomedical Books
New York

For permission to use material from this book please contact us:
Telephone 631-231-7269; Fax 631-231-8175
Web Site: http://www.novapublishers.com

Library of Congress Cataloging-in-Publication Data

Iencean, Stefan Mircea.
Intracranial hypertension / Stefan Mircea Iencean, Alexandru Vladimir Ciurea.
p. ; cm.
Includes bibliographical references and index.
ISBN 978-1-60741-862-7 (hardcover)
1. Intracranial hypertension. I. Ciurea, A. V. II. Title.
[DNLM: 1. Intracranial Hypertension--physiopathology. 2. Intracranial Hypertension--diagnosis. WL 203 I22i 2009]
RC386.2.I36 2009
616.1'32--dc22

2009019830

Published by Nova Science Publishers, Inc. ✢ New York

Contents

Preface

Intracranial hypertension (ICH) is a fundamental issue of neurology and neurosurgery. The skull is a rigid structure. Brain, blood and cerebrospinal fluid are incompressible and according to the "Monroe-Kellie doctrine" an increase in one constituent or an expanding mass within the skull results in an increase in intracranial pressure. In these conditions, ICH dominates the neurologic pathology and the cranio-cerebral neurosurgical pathology.

Any important headache refractory to treatment associated with morning explosive vomiting will outline better the ICH syndrome. The finding of the papillar edema shows the breakdown of the compensating possibilities of various intracranial compartments in case of developing of an expanding mass, and especially the severity of this syndrome that reaches a critical point with vital involvement. In the event of additional focal neurologic signs (ataxia, motor impairment, cranial nerve palsy, speech impairment etc), the intracranial hypertension syndrome certainly includes an intracranial lesion.

The authors attract attention of this cardinal point wherein the ICH phenomena could acquire sometimes quickly a bad evolution. The authors also insist about the need of a fast and full diagnosis of ICH syndrome and most of all about its pathogeny.

The present monography achieves an unitary, synthetic and coherent approach of this thorny problem - intracranial hypertension, also offering an original pathogenic classification.

The proposed etiopathogenic classification includes perfect differentiated elements in the generation of ICH: parenchimatous ICH with cerebral intrinsic etiopathogenesis; vascular ICH secondary to the cerebral circulation disorders; ICH caused by CSF dynamic disorders and idiopathic ICH. In relation to the idiopathic ICH, it can have many possible causes, but the pathogenesis is the same - the changing of the brain blood barrier, which determines the increase of intraparenchimatous cerebral fluid with respective clinical consequences. It is possible that future research will relieve other mechanisms in the pathogeny of idiopathic ICH.

Finally, the authors insist upon the importance of ICH and its diagnosis, which has to be as correct as possible and in short time, and of the treatment for each type of intracranial hypertension.This work addresses to all specialties in medicine, especially to neurologists, neurosurgeons, intensive care neurologists, ophthalmologists, otolaryngologists etc.

Stefan M Iencean, MD, PhD
AV Ciurea, MD, PhD

Chapter I

Intracranial Hypertension General Approach

Intracranial hypertension represents the increase in the intracranial pressure (ICP) due to the disturbance of the regulating mechanisms for intracranial pressure. It is caused by the intrinsic changes in the volumes of the intracranial compartments: brain parenchyma, cerebrospinal fluid and blood content, and/or by the adding of a pathological volume.

The descriptive classification of the intracranial hypertension (ICH) has been replaced by an etio-pathogenic classification with four main groups:

- parenchymatous intracranial hypertension,
- vascular intracranial hypertension,
- intracranial hypertension caused by the disorders of the cerebro-spinal fluid dynamics,
- idiopathic intracranial hypertension.

The evolution of the intracranial hypertension has three stages:

- the increase in the intracranial pressure is a warning signal at first;
- then the ICP increase exceeds the critical value generating the ICH syndrome
- compensatory mechanisms may no longer block the evolution towards the acute stage.

1. General Approach and Short History

Intracranial hypertension (ICH) is a fundamental issue of neurology and neurosurgery, having important implications in other medical-surgical specialties since it may be a complication in the evolution of many disorders of internal medicine, endocrinology, ophthalmology, obstetrics, etc.

Intracranial hypertension represents the increase in intracranial pressure (ICP) due to disorders of the regulating mechanisms for intracranial pressure. It is caused by the intrinsic changes in the volumes of the intracranial compartments: brain parenchyma, cerebrospinal fluid and blood content, and/or by the adding of a pathological volume. [5,10]

At first, the increase in intracranial pressure is caused by changes in the volume-pressure relations in correlation with time (the speed of occurrence and the duration of changes), which is induced by various etiologies. Afterwards, the intracranial hypertension causes physio-pathological disorders which cause specific changes to the endocranial structures, and, therefore, the subsequent ICP increase is accompanied by its own symptomatology.

Thus, intracranial hypertension is a sign of the causal illness and, concomitantly, it constitutes a syndrome evolving in parallel to the initial illness, or it may seem to have an independent evolution. In relation to its causal mechanism, intracranial hypertension is and it may remain a symptom (increased intracranial pressure), or it evolves as a syndrome (increased intracranial pressure associated with other signs and symptoms). There are ICP values that are considered to be at the normal limit or moderately increased values, which do not induce evolutionary physio-pathological mechanisms by themselves. The subsequent evolution of ICH as a syndrome results from the very transformation of the initial ICP increase into a pathogenic mechanism and from the progression of the characteristic symptoms, whose intensity may exceed even the symptomatology of the initial illness.

When the increased intracranial pressure represents the cause of other disorders having their own development, it is correlated with the limits of the compensation capacities of pressure increase. This is the stage when the occurred symptomatology becomes specific and the intracranial hypertension turns into an illness with an individual evolution. [2,5]

As far as its evolution is concerned, ICH may have a different nosologic classification: the increased ICP as an initial symptom, then ICH is the syndrome manifested in several illnesses, and it may be a separate illness afterwards. From the perspective of the evolutionary stage (sign, syndrome or illness), the etiopathogeny – physiopathology relation is modified, and the therapeutic priorities are differentiated. Intracranial hypertension as a syndrome corresponds to the period when compensating intracranial pressure increases is possible, while ICH as an illness is generated by exceeding the compensating capacities of the increases in intracranial hypertension; therefore, ICH as an illness is the decompensated syndrome of intracranial hypertension. In ICH syndrome, the causal illness must be identified and treated, and, when ICH has become an illness, the first measures are decreasing the intracranial pressure and then, or concomitantly, identifying and treating the initial cause of the ICP.

In relation to the type of evolution, intracranial hypertension can be:

- intracranial hypertension in initial stage, only with an increased ICP,
- intracranial hypertension in compensated stage; this is the ICH syndrome,
- intracranial hypertension as an illness, by a decompensation of the ICH syndrome or as an acute form since the beginning.[4,5,10]

From an evolution perspective, the ICH syndrome may be stationary or it may evolve in two ways: a progressive aggravation occurs until decompensation and transformation into an illness, or the evolution is remissive, under treatment or spontaneous.

The historical evolution of knowledge on intracranial hypertension has had a first long stage of clinical accumulation, underlining the major clinical symptoms and establishing the relation between the presence of ICH and the existence of a process that replaces the intracranial space, especially a tumor process. Afterwards, it has been noticed that ICH may also exist in the absence of an expansive intracranial lesion, and these situations have been designated by the phrase pseudotumor cerebri.

The invention of the ophthalmoscope by von Helmholtz in 1851 was followed by the study of the optic fundus in neurological illnesses (von Graeffe, Albutt, Jackson etc.) and the confirmation of the existence of the papillary edema in intracranial hypertension. In 1866, Lyden measures the intracranial pressure by a trephine hole; in the same year, Knoll records certain charts of the cerebrospinal fluid pressure, and, in 1870 Duret notices a clinical aggravation on experimental animals (dogs), who have experienced an intracranial introduction of fluids by the trephine hole, which proves that the increase in the intracranial pressure is associated to the decrease in the cerebral blood perfusion.

At the end of the 19th century, the lumbar puncture is introduced for the study of the cerebrospinal fluid composition and pressure in neurological illnesses (Quincke). The progressive discovery of new investigating means of the nervous system throughout the 20th century: ventriculography, carotid angiography, scintigraphic exploration, intracranial pressure monitoring, computerized cerebral tomography, nuclear magnetic resonance imaging, tomography with positron emission, SPECT, etc., have all led to more knowledge about intracranial hypertension and the identification of the most efficient therapy for it.

2. Classification of Intracranial Hypertension

The ICH classification in two main groups had been accepted for a long time: intracranial hypertension that had occurred in intracranial expansive processes, and the pseudo-tumor intracranial hypertension, which occurs in other illnesses than the intracranial expansive processes, and which is also known by the name of pseudotumor cerebri.

Nowadays, there is a descriptive presentation of ICH, according to which it is divided into two groups: secondary intracranial hypertension, when the increase in the intracranial pressure is generated by an obvious cause (tumor, cerebral venous thrombosis, meningitis, etc.) and the idiopathic intracranial hypertension, with no noticeable cause. [1,5,11,12]

The descriptive classification of the clinical forms of intracranial hypertension includes:

1 Intracranial hypertension caused by a tumor

The appearance and the evolution of the ICH syndrome depend on the location of the tumor and the expansion of the tumor. Intracranial benign tumors have a slow rate of volume increase and the neurological syndrome appears gradually, while the ICH syndrome may appear rather late. Malignant tumors have a rapid developing rate and the neurological syndrome appears precociously.

Cerebral glioma with a reduced degree of malignity: ICH syndrome with papillary edema appears more rarely because, quite frequently, the tumor location does not affect the circulation of the cerebro-spinal fluid, and because the dominating symptoms appear before the increase in the tumor volume, which may generate signs of intracranial hypertension.

Cerebral glioma with an increased degree of malignity: the mechanisms that lead to the apparition of the ICH syndrome are local parenchymatous as a compression on the neighbouring structures or on the circulation paths of the cerebro-spinal fluid, and diffuse intracranial mechanisms caused by the increase in intracranial pressure due to the tumor volume.

Cerebral metastases are accompanied by an important brain edema, and intracranial hypertension is frequently present.

Intracranial benign tumors have a slow growing rate and their clinic evolution is represented by the focal neurological syndromes, and the ICH syndrome appears later. Most frequently the ICH syndrome appears by blocking the circulation of the cerebro-spinal fluid.

2 Intracranial hypertension in extending non-traumatic and non-tumor intracranial lesions

The occurrence and the development of the ICH syndrome in cases of hydatid cyst or in extending infectious lesions (cerebral abscess, subdural or extradural empyema) depend on the location of the lesion relative to the circulation of the cerebro-spinal fluid and the involvement of the venous circulation.

3 Intracranial hypertension in cranio-cerebral traumatisms

The ICH syndrome and its clinical deterioration are caused by the mechanisms and the speed with which traumatic endo-cranial lesions are produced. Primary or secondary traumatic lesions bring about the increase in the intracranial pressure by increasing the endo-cranial volume due to: a supplementary volume added by a traumatic haematoma, by a brain edema or by the increase in the volume of the cerebro-spinal fluid.

4 Intracranial hypertension in congenital malformations

Cranio-cerebral and cranio-spinal malformations and cranio-synostoses: Dandy-Walker, Chiari type II, Crouzon illness, etc., cause the occurrence of intracranial hypertension by means of disorders of the cerebro-spinal fluid circulation.

5 Intracranial hypertension in hypertensive encephalopathy

Hypertensive encephalopathy is defined by the clinical presentation of intracranial hypertension induced by an acute episode of high blood pressure, which leads to an increase in the volume of the cerebral parenchyma due to the brain swelling and / or brain edema.

6 Intracranial hypertension in ischemic cerebral-vascular illness

Wide ischemic cerebral lesions are accompanied by a brain edema with brain herniation and by an increase in the ICP. The cerebral infarction extended by intracranial hypertension is caused by the occlusion or the stenosis of a cerebral great artery. The extended ischemic infarction of the Sylvian artery has been named the malign infarct of the Sylvian artery due to the increased mortality. A generalized brain ischemia occurs in the post-resuscitation syndrome, when the blood flow disorder covers the entire brain by a complete ischemia throughout the cardiac arrest, followed by reperfusion disorders.

7 Intracranial hypertension in cerebral venous thrombosis

Cerebral venous thrombosis reduces the returning venous flow; a venous stasis is produced and the brain blood circulation is slowed down. The symptomatology is generated by the initial causal lesion; then neurological focal symptoms appear, related to the progression of the venous thrombosis, as well as symptoms caused by the increase in the intracranial pressure.

8 Intracranial hypertension in obstructive internal hydrocephalus

Intracranial hypertension is caused by circulation disorders of the cerebro-spinal fluid.

The circulation of the cerebro-spinal fluid is blocked by: Sylvius aqueduct stenosis; intra-ventricular expansive processes; the extrinsic blockage of the ventricular system by para-ventricular lesions; the obstruction of communication with sub-arachnoid cisterns.

Hydrocephalus symptoms vary according to how long ago the illness had appeared, the way the hydrocephalus progresses and its individual characteristics. The evolution of the ICH syndrome is fast and it may lead to decompensated intracranial hypertension [6,8]

9 Intracranial hypertension due to the decrease in the resorption of the CSF

Intracranial hypertension is caused by the decrease in the resorption of the cerebro-spinal fluid due to various causes influencing the resorption mechanisms: in acute meningitis, in subarachnoid hemorrhage, in brain trauma etc. The cerebro-spinal fluid gathers in the ventricular system and a communicating hydrocephalus occurs with an intracranial hypertension syndrome.

10 Intracranial hypertension of toxic etiology (endogenous or exogenous).

It appears in the absence of an expanding intracranial lesion, in the absence of a brain trauma, without vascular etiology etc. It is caused by a diffuse cerebral suffering, caused by endogenous or exogenous toxic elements, and it often has an acute beginning.

The posterior reversible encephalopathy syndrome (PRES) has two etiologies: hypertensive encephalopathy, which includes the syndrome into the intracranial hypertension group with various causes of the high blood pressure episode, and the toxic cause due to the action of several immuno-suppressors or cytostatics, which includes the syndromes having this etiology into the intracranial hypertension group of toxic cause.

The intracranial hypertension caused by a fulminate hepatic insufficiency [hepatic encephalopathy] probably has a multifactor etiopathogeny via the combination of the cytotoxic brain edema due to the intra-astrocytary accumulation of glutamine, and by the brain swelling caused by vascular dilatation, and the increase in the cerebral blood volume due to inflammation, glutamate and the toxic elements due to the hepatic dysfunction.

11 Idiopathic intracranial hypertension

The idiopathic intracranial hypertension is characterized by the increase in intracranial pressure in the absence of any of: an expansive intracranial process, hydrocephalus, an intracranial infection, thrombosis of the dural venous sinuses, or hypertensive encephalopathy. The idiopathic intracranial hypertension partially corresponds to the old designation of pseudotumor cerebri. The diagnosis of idiopathic intracranial hypertension may be given only after the measurement of the intracranial pressure and after a complete neuro-imagistic exploration.[1,3,7,9]

Depending on the etiology and on the pathogenic mechanism that causes the disorder in the volume-intracranial pressure relation, and based on the variation of the intracranial pressure over time, there is now an etiopathogenic classification of the intracranial hypertension, which includes both the etiopathogenic mechanisms and the clinical data (Iencean 2001, revised 2003).

Many of the previous observations and findings of other authors have foreseen the following systematization. [4,5,12]

1. Parenchymatous Intracranial Hypertension

It occurs in the extending intracranial processes (cerebral tumors, intracranial haematoma, cerebral abscesses, etc.), in the traumatic brain edema, in the cerebral ischemia with hypotoxic brain edema, in general intoxications with neurotoxins (endogenous or exogenous) etc. The primary cerebral etiology is known and it causes changes of the intracranial volume; the brain edema appears afterwards and it evolves in parallel to the increase in the ICP. The parenchymatous lesion initially appears as a result of the intrinsic cerebral etiology and of the primary modifications in the intracranial volume (expansive, compressive, hypotoxic or traumatic brain edema). The parenchymatous intracranial hypertension may have a complete development to its acute form with a brain stem ischemia or brain herniation.

2. Vascular Intracranial Hypertension

The ICP increase is caused by disorders of the cerebral or extra-cerebral blood circulation. The increased volume of the brain parenchyma in vascular ICH is produced by a brain edema or by an increase in the cerebral blood volume (brain swelling). The brain edema and/or the congestive cerebral parenchyma will lead to an increased intracranial pressure. The increase in the cerebral sanguine volume occurs when there is an increased intracranial arterial blood supply or a decreased blockage of the venous drainage. When the venous drainage is reduced, there is also a decrease in the resorption of the cerebro-spinal fluid. The "congestive brain" aspect is caused by the increase in the intra-cerebral blood volume, and the volume-intracranial pressure conflict occurs. At the level of the structure represented by the nervous parenchyma – vascular capillary, two types of changes happen, which may be separate or have an evolutionary connection between them: the stage of a brain edema, due to water accumulation in the parenchyma, and the stage of brain swelling (congestive brain), with an increase in the volume of the cerebral parenchyma due to vascular dilatation.

The vascular intracranial hypertension appears in:

- cerebral illnesses: by affecting the venous return and blocking the cerebro-spinal fluid absorption in cerebral venous thrombosis, thrombosis of superior sagittal sinus, cerebral thrombophlebites, mastoiditis ("otitic hydrocephalus", described by Symonds– thrombosis of venous sinuses, secondary to oto-mastoiditis) etc., by slowing down or decreasing the venous flow in the superior longitudinal sinus in the arterio-venous shunt in certain types of intra-cerebral vascular malformations, especially Galien vein aneurysms, or by decreasing the blood feeding in brain ischemias with secondary ischemic brain edema, as in the ischemic stroke caused by the occlusion or stenosis of the big cerebral vessels, with a serious form of malignant ischemic infarction within the territory of the middle cerebral artery (massive Sylvian infarction).
- extra-cerebral illnesses: hypertensive encephalopathy with brain swelling and with extra-cellular hydrostatic brain edema (by ultra-filtration); in the cervical or thoracic venous blockage.

The vascular intracranial hypertension usually develops only until the occurrence of a complete ICH syndrome; but, sometimes, it may develop until the occurrence of the acute form of ICH due to secondary disorders of the cerebral blood circulation. In the case of the massive ischemic infarction within the territory of the middle cerebral artery, the brain edema occurs quickly, it is extensive and the intracranial hypertension has an acute development, with a mortality of up to 80% of the cases.

3. Intracranial Hypertension Due to Disorders of the Cerebro-Spinal Fluid Dynamics

The dynamics of the cerebro-spinal fluid includes the circulation of the cerebro-spinal fluid from the time of its creation at the level of the choroid plexuses, and up to its passage into the venous circulation.

The dynamic disorders of the cerebro-spinal fluid may be:

- circulation disorders of the cerebro-spinal fluid from its creation until resorption, and

- disorders in the passage of the cerebro-spinal fluid in the venous drainage system (resorption).

The circulation disorders of the cerebro-spinal fluid occur when there is an obstacle in the fluid itinerary (ventricular system, magna cistern, basal cisterns) due to the existence of a ventricular or para-ventricular tumor, intra-ventricular hemorrhage, or obstruction of various causes of the Sylvius aqueduct. A dilatation of the segments of the ventricular system occurs (those that are supra-adjacent to the obstruction), while the clinical presentation and the evolution are related to the obstructive internal hydrocephalus.

The resorption disorders of the cerebro-spinal fluid occur due to the lesions of the anatomic structures that provide the passage of the cerebro-spinal fluid from the sub-arachnoid spaces into the venous drainage system in acute meningitis, in sub-arachnoid hemorrhage, in meningitis carcinomatosis, in sarcoidosis chronic meningitis, etc. A thickening of the leptomeninx occurs, blocking the Pachioni's arachnoid granulations, and decreasing the absorption of the cerebro-spinal fluid. The cerebro-spinal fluid accumulates in the sub-arachnoid spaces and in the ventricular system, leading to a communicating hydrocephalus, with a peri-ventricular hydrocephalic brain edema and with an intracranial hypertension syndrome, which is usually a sub-acute one. The clinical presentation and the increase in the intracranial pressure adds the intracranial hypertension syndrome in cases of cerebro-spinal fluid circulation obstruction.

4. Idiopathic Intracranial Hypertension

This form of ICH has also been designated as pseudotumor cerebri, essential or cryptogenic ICH, a terminology that is outdated. The etiology could not be established. It occurs in endocrine illnesses, metabolic disorders or various hematological illnesses etc. Not long ago, physio-pathological mechanisms were thought to include various disorders of the cerebro-spinal fluid secretion and absorption, so that the increase in the ICP is secondary to the decrease in the cerebrospinal fluid absorption without the occurence of hydrocephalus (this theory is also sustained by the efficiency of the lombo-peritoneal shunt). Moreover, the brain edema could be caused by the so-called non-specific “associated factors”, which lead to the ICP increase, without the possibility of establishing an etiological relation.

The most probable current pathogenic hypothesis about the idiopathic intracranial hypertension is based on the dynamics of the intracranial fluid circuits that allow maintaining the self-regulation of the cerebral circulation and of the cerebral blood flow. In idiopathic ICH there are various pathologic conditions that cause progressive damage to the brain blood barrier with a hyper-production of interstitial fluid and the occurrence of the extra-cellular brain edema. Usually, the cerebro-spinal fluid is produce as normal, and the increased pressure from the cerebral parenchyma is equalized by the pressure of the cerebro-spinal fluid by means of increased exchanges from the interstitial fluid towards the cerebro-spinal fluid at the pial trans-cerebral and trans-ependymal level. The increase in the fluid pressure is followed by the increase in the resorption of the cerebro-spinal fluid and by a rapid venous efflux, so that the increased intracranial pressure does not affect the cerebral circulation, which is maintained within the normal limits. The trans-ependymal and the trans-pial circuit of the interstitial fluid towards the cerebro-spinal fluid represents and efficient compensatory mechanism when the intracranial pressure increases gradually and allows cerebral circulatory self-regulation.

Therefore, idiopathic ICH occurs due to the impact on the brain blood barrier, via various causes that are not established yet, with a hyper-production of interstitial fluid and an extra-cellular brain edema, with increased exchanges from the interstitial fluid towards the cerebro-spinal fluid at the trans-ependymal and trans-pial level; an increased resorption of the cerebro-spinal fluid occurs and there is a rapid venous efflux.

The idiopathic ICH develops into an incomplete ICH syndrome, despite the increased ICP values and the presence of the papillary edema.

The established causes for certain forms of ICH–considered idiopathic will probably include them into one of the ICH forms with a known etiology: vascular, meningeal or parenchymatous.

The ICH syndrome may also appear as a form of transition between these four forms of ICH, or it may be induced by several concomitant pathogenic mechanisms of the brain edema in: bacillary meningo-encephalitis, neoplasia, hydro-electrolytic disorders, diabetic keto-acidosis, PRES, etc.

The comparison between the ICH forms underlines the existing differences very clearly (table 1).

The decompensation in parenchymatous intracranial hypertension is more rapid and it happens at lower values than in idiopathic ICH due to the existence of the pressure differences between the cranio-spinal compartments and the occurrence of the cerebral circulation disorders with a decrease in the cerebral perfusion pressure in parenchymatous ICH.

The increased critical values of the intracranial pressure, the period of ICP increase and the duration of the ICP action are the main parameters that control the intracranial biomechanical fluid stability, and which cause the pressure and circulatory decompensation. The state of clinical instability is happens because of the increase in values of the intracranial pressure and it appears when the increased ICP action time is longer than the compensation cerebral capacity.

The pressure-time fluctuation defines the pressure increase relative to the action duration of the increased intracranial pressure, which induces the self-regulation disorder of the cerebral blood circulation. The limit decompensation conditions appear when the duration of the increased ICP action is longer than the period corresponding to the same pressure values in the pressure compensation situation, or the ICP values are higher than the ICP values corresponding to the same duration of action.

The development of intracranial hypertension has three stages and it overcomes the critical ICP moments the moment it passes to the next stage:

a) at first, the ICP increase is an alarm signal;
b) afterwards, the ICP increase exceeds the critical value for the occurrence of the ICH syndrome; the ICH syndrome evolves depending on the existing etiology and on the

maintenance of self-regulation of the cerebral blood circulation. The compensatory mechanisms may stop the pressure-time fluctuation.

c) finally, the acute critical ICP values lead to the alteration of the circulatory self-regulation, and the compensatory mechanisms can no longer stop the development towards the acute stage.

The first and the second stages are reversible, and the third stage corresponds to a phase of maximum instability when the decompensation with clinical aggravation occurs via brain stem ischemia or brain herniation, which generates irreversible cerebral lesions.

The etiological temporal relation classifies the causes of the intracranial hypertension into:

- acute causes that lead to the acute increase in the intracranial pressure and the rapid installation of the ICH syndrome, and which include brain trauma, acute ischemic lesions or intra-cerebral hemorrhage; exogenous or endogenous intoxications with the rapid formation of the brain edema, as well as infections such as encephalitis or meningitis which may lead to ICH too;
- chronic causes, which produce the progressive increase in the intracranial pressure and the belated decompensation of the ICH; they include many of the intracranial tumors with slow evolution, progressive blockage of the cerebro-spinal fluid circulation, the chronic subdural haematoma, the idiopathic ICH etc.

Table 1. Main characteristics of the intracranial hypertension forms

		ICH by dynamics disorders of the CSF		
Parenchymatous ICH	**Vascular ICH**	**By obstruction**	**Meningeal ICH**	**Idiopathic ICH**
Known etiology: cerebral lesion	Etiology: cerebral or general vascular illness	Known etiology: circulation obstruction of the cerebro-spinal fluid	Known etiology: meningeal inflammation, etc.	Etiology not mentioned or various non-specific factors: "associated factors"
Present brain edema (cyto-toxic, vasogenic) perifocal / sectorial	Present brain edema (vasogenic) sectorial or generalized	Obstructive hydrocephalus with peri-ventricular or generalized edema	Communicating hydrocephalus with peri-ventricular or generalized edema	Brain edema, balanced by an intra-ventricular ICP
Rapid ICP increase	Moderate ICP increase	Rapid ICP increase	Moderate ICP increase	Very slow ICP increase
Critical ICP value ≈ 20 mm Hg	Critical ICP value ≈ 20 mm Hg	Critical ICP value ≈ 20 mm Hg	Critical ICP value ≈ 20 mm Hg	High ICP values ≈ 60-80 mm Hg
ICP differences between cerebro-spinal compartments	Usual, without ICP differences between cerebro-spinal compartments	ICP differences between cerebro-spinal compartments	There are no ICP differences between cerebro-spinal compartments	Constantly increased ICP in all the cerebro-spinal compartments
The increased ICP reduces the self-regulation of the cerebral circulation	The vascular illness reduces the self-regulation of the cerebral circulation	The increased ICP reduces the self-regulation of the cerebral circulation	The inflammatory vasculitis may affect the self-regulation of the cerebral circulation	The self-regulation of the cerebral circulation is maintained, with an intense absorption of the cerebro-spinal fluid and of the parenchymatous interstitial fluid

Table 1. (Continued)

Parenchymatous ICH	Vascular ICH	ICH by dynamics disorders of the CSF By obstruction	Meningeal ICH	Idiopathic ICH
Short duration of action for increased ICP	Long duration of the pressure-time fluctuation	Short duration of action for increased ICP	Variable duration of the pressure-time fluctuation	Very long duration of the pressure-time fluctuation
Complete development into ~~a~~ decompensated ICH by cerebral hernia, cerebral stem ischemia	Usual development into ICH syndrome	Complete development into decompensated ICH	Etiology dependent development, usually into a complete or incomplete ICH syndrome	Development into an incomplete ICH syndrome. Discordance: minimum clinic compared to a high ICP and the papillary edema; possible decrease in visual acuity
Etiological treatment: often neurosurgical	Symptomatic or etiologic treatment; rarely decompressive craniectomy in massif, hemispheric ischemic infarct	Neurosurgical treatment: etiologic or ventricular drainage	Symptomatic and/or etiological treatment; sometimes, ventricular drainage in acute hydrocephalus	Symptomatic treatment of the "associated factors" too; lombo-peritoneal shunt, decompression of the optic nerve

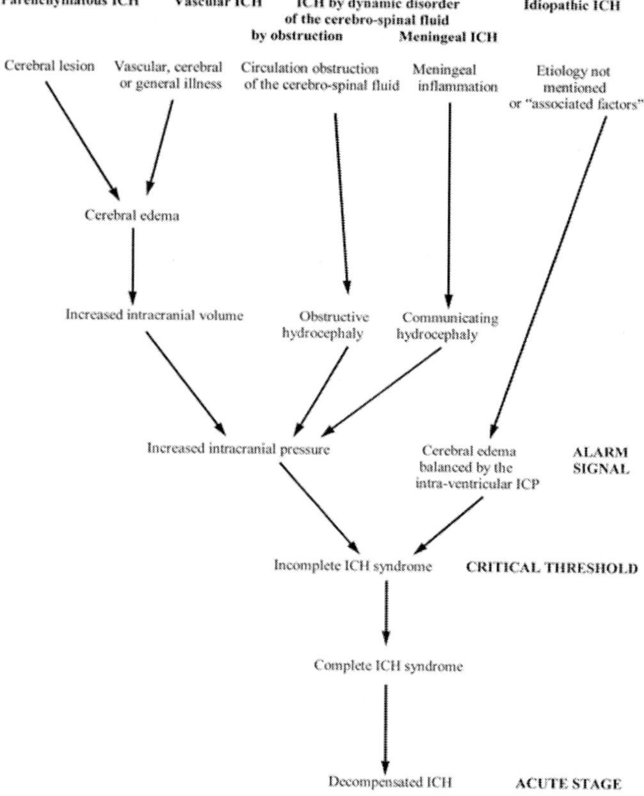

Figure 1. Etiological and evolutionary chart of intracranial hypertension forms

References

[1] Digre KB, Nakamoto BK, Warner JE, Langeberg WJ, Baggaley SK, Katz BJ.A Comparison of Idiopathic Intracranial Hypertension With and Without Papilledema.Headache. 2009 ;49, 2:185-193.

[2] Frank JI, Rosengart AJ . Intracranial pressure : monitoring and managenment, In Wood LDH, Hall JB, Schmidt GA. Principles of critical care, McGraw-Hill Professional, 2005, 1007 -1024

[3] Goodwin J. Recent developments in idiopathic intracranial hypertension (IIH), Seminars in Ophthalmology, 2003, 18, 4 : 181 – 189

[4] Iencean St M. A new classification and a synergetical pattern in intracranial hypertension Medical Hypotheses , 2002 ;58,2 :159-63.

[5] Iencean St M. Pattern of increased intracranial pressure and classification of intracranial hypertension. Journal of Medical Sciences, 2004, 4, 1 :52- 58

[6] Johnston IH, Duff J, Jacobson EE, Fagan E . Asymptomatic Intracranial Hypertension in Disorders of CSF Circulation in Childhood - Treated and Untreated, Pediatric Neurosurgery ,2001;34:63-72

[7] Johnston I, Owler B, Pickard J . The Pseudotumor Cerebri Syndrome: Pseudotumor Cerebri, Idiopathic Intracranial Hypertension, Benign Intracranial Hypertension and Related Conditions, Cambridge University Press, 2007

[8] Lee HS, Yoon SH. Hypothesis for lateral ventricular dilatation in communicating hydrocephalus: New understanding of the Monro-Kellie hypothesis in the aspect of cardiac energy transfer through arterial blood flow.Med Hypotheses, 2009 ;72, 2:174-7

[9] Lehman CA. Idiopathic intracranial hypertension within the ICF model: a review of the literature. J Neurosci Nurs. 2003 ;35,5:263-9

[10] Marmarou A. The pathophysiology of brain edema and elevated intracranial pressure. Cleve Clin J Med. 2004 ;71 Suppl 1:S6-8.

[11] Penson, R.; Allen, R. Intracranial hypertension: condition monitoring, simulation and time domain analysis, Engineering Science and Education Journal, 1999, 8, 1: 33- 40

[12] Santiago ME, Cornett JJ. Raised cerebrospinal fluid pressure headache, In Goadsby PJ, Silberstein SD, Dodick D. Chronic daily headache for clinicians, PMPH-USA, 2005, 167 – 182

Chapter II

Introduction to Anatomy and Physiology

Intracranial hypertension (ICH) refers to the pathological modifications of the brain and to the clinical manifestations occurred due to the disorder of the volume-intracranial pressure relation. The skull (neurocranium) communicates with the spinal channel at the level of the occipital hole and the nervous continuity and the continuity of the cerebrospinal fluid are extremely important in the ICH evolution (the involvement of the cerebellar amygdales in acute ICH, the drainage of the lumbar cerebrospinal fluid in idiopathic ICH etc.). Thus, although ICH refers to the endocranial segment of the central nervous system, its evolution and complications may also affect the spinal segment, especially the fluid component (CSF).

1. The Cranio-Spinal Space

The central nervous system (CNS) is covered by the meninges and it is located in the cranio-spinal space. Dura mater is attached to the internal skull and the endocranial volume corresponds to the volume provided by the cranial dura mater. At the spine, dura mater usually continues to the level of S2 vertebra, and it is in partial contact only with the anterior wall of the spinal channel. [3,4,8]

The cerebral cranium (neurocranium) contains the encephalon and the meningeal layers.

The neurocranium includes the skull-cap or calvaria and the base (basis). The neurocranium is made of four odd bones: frontal, ethmoid, sphenoid and occipital, as well as two pairs of bones: the temporal bones and the parietal bones. The cranium of a new-born child is characterized by a small viscerocranium compared to the neurocranium. Ossification is not complete at birth, and at the intersection of the sutures, there are areas of non-ossified conjunctive tissue, called fontanelles, which correspond to the membranous stage of bone ossification. The anterior fontanelle has a rhomboidal shape and it is placed on the median line at the frontal-parietal intersection (the median intersection of the frontal and sagittal sutures and the two halves of the coronary suture). Usually, it closes up by the age of two years old.

The posterior fontanelle is triangular and it is located at the posterior end of the sagittal suture, between the parietal and occipital bones, and it usually closes during the second month of life.

Bilaterally, there are the anterior sphenoidal fontanelle and the posterior mastoid fontanelle.

The cranium development includes three stages:

- the first period includes the first seven years and it is characterized by a significant cranial growth;
- the second period starts at the age of seven and lasts until the beginning of the puberty period; it is a period of relative stagnation;
- the third period starts at the beginning of the puberty period (13-14 years old) until the bone growth stops (19-23 years old).

The cranial sutures close up as they turn into synostoses; the coronal suture closes between 11-20 years old, while the sagittal suture closes between 20-30 years old; the lambdoid suture is the last to close up or it may remain open. There are gender differences related to the size of the cranium: man's average cranial capacity is bigger than the woman's by 10 %, with variations included between 1250 cm^3 and 1500 cm^3. The woman's smaller size has no connection to the cerebral development, but it is proportional to the dimensions of the body.

The cranial aspect is individually different; the relation between the maximum diameter / maximum length represents the cephalic index (CI), and it allows the establishment of three cranial morphological types:

- the brachycephalic or "short-headed" with the cephalic index (CI) > 80 ,
- the mesocephalic or "medium-headed" with CI: 75-80 and
- the dolichocephalic or "long-headed" with CI < 75 .

These individual physiological variations are not related to the occurrence of the intracranial hypertension in various pathological situations.

Endocranial dura mater is different of the spinal dura mater : dura mater adheres to the internal skull and at the level of the spinal channel dura mater does not adhere, but it is closer to the anterior wall and it usually ends at the level of the S2 vertebra. [10,15]

Dura mater presents a conjunctive-fibrous structure and it is considered to be slightly extensible. The extradural space is intracranially reduced, and it is represented by the extradural compartments laterally to the Turkish saddle, where there are numerous veins beside the internal carotid artery, nerves and a bit of adipose tissue (an area known as "cavernous sinus"), and it does not allow a significant dural expansion.

At the level of the spinal channel, the extradural space is bigger on the posterior-lateral and the inferior sides. The dural elasticity is reduced, but an expansion may be achieved by compressing the spinal extradural venous plexuses. The study of the volume / subdural pressure variation has revealed an increased compliance (the compliance is the volume variation per pressure unit) for the spinal dural sac, and a decreased compliance for the cranial dura mater. This means that the spinal dura-mater presents a certain degree of elasticity, therefore, the spinal dural sac may extend, accepting a supplementary volume with no increase in the intracranial/subdural pressure. Since the dural structure is the same, from a cranial and a spinal perspective, the difference of dural extensibility also seems to depend on the existence and the size of the extradural space.

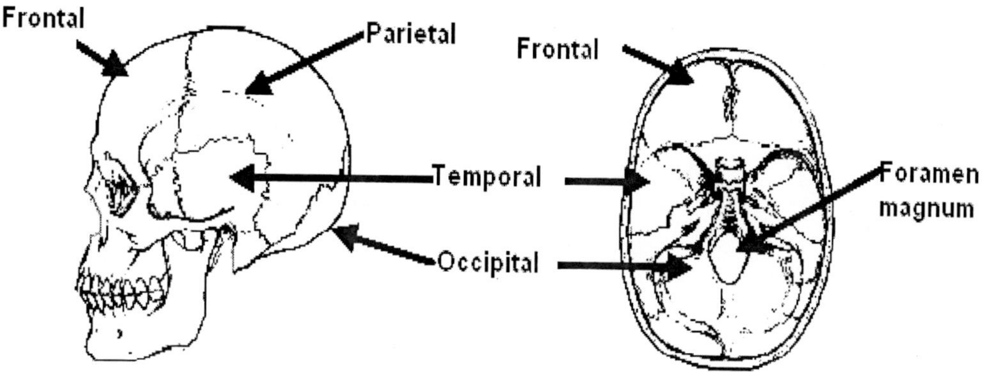

Figure 2. Normal cranium, lateral image, and skull base, endocranial image

The cranial dura mater presents prolongations that divide the endocranial space, and which separate different parts of the encephalon and these are maintained in a relatively stable position.

Thus the tent of the cerebellum or tentorium cerebelli is a prolongation of the dura mater, which is located between the encephalon and the cerebellum, and it establishes a superior limit to the posterior cerebral fosse or the cerebellar fosse. It originates in the level of the clinoid apophyses, having a free anterior concave margin named incisura tentorii. The external convex margin is adherent and it represents a continuation of the endocranial dura mater at the level of the occipital transversal groove and of the occipital protuberance. On the external margin of the cerebellum tent, along the transversal occipital groove, the transversal dural sinus has a bilateral location, and it is a continuation of the superior sagittal sinus and of the right sinus. The scythe of the brain or falx cerebri is a median supra-tentorial prolongation of the sagittally oriented dura mater. It is fixed on an anterior spot to the crista galli apophysis, it has the shape of a scythe, and its width progressively increases in the posterior direction, where it is fixed on the median edge of the cerebellum tent. The inferior margin is concave and free, and it penetrates between the two cerebral hemispheres, near the callous corpus, and it contains the inferior sagittal sinus, while the fixing base on the cerebellum tent contains the right venous sinus. The superior margin has a median insertion on dura mater, which has a frontal-parietal convexity to the internal occipital protuberance, limiting the superior sagittal sinus.

These endocranial dural prolongations together with the rachial dural sac divide the cranial spinal space in four compartments:

- two supra-tentorial compartments, each of them corresponding to a cerebral hemisphere, partially separated by the brain scythe;

- a sub-tentorial compartment, which is separated from the cerebral hemispheres by the tentorium and communicates with the supra-tentorial compartments by means of the space that is limited by the free margin of the cerebellum tent and with the spinal channel by means of the occipital hole;
- a spinal, cylindrical compartment, representing the spinal dural sac.

Based on the location of a particular pathologic process, these compartments are involved in the occurrence of certain pressure differences that may cause movements of the cerebral structures, which represents a cerebral herniation.

Under the dura mater and separated from it by means of a capillary space (fissure), there is the arachnoid, which forms the leptomeninges together with pia mater. The arachnoid presents an areolar structure and, together with pia mater, it sets the limits of the sub-arachnoid space containing the cerebrospinal fluid. The subarachnoid space has certain larger areas that represent subarachnoid cisterns or lakes.

From an endocranial perspective, the most important ones are the cerebellomedullary cistern, the ponto-medullary cistern, the basal cistern etc.; at the pouch of the spinal dural sac, in the lumbar region, there is the inferior medullar lake or the lumbar cistern. The sub-arachnoid space is prolonged along certain cranial nerves, around the radices of the spinal nerves and through the Virchow-Robin perivascular spaces, which surround the arterioles and the venules, and penetrates into the depth of the nervous tissue.

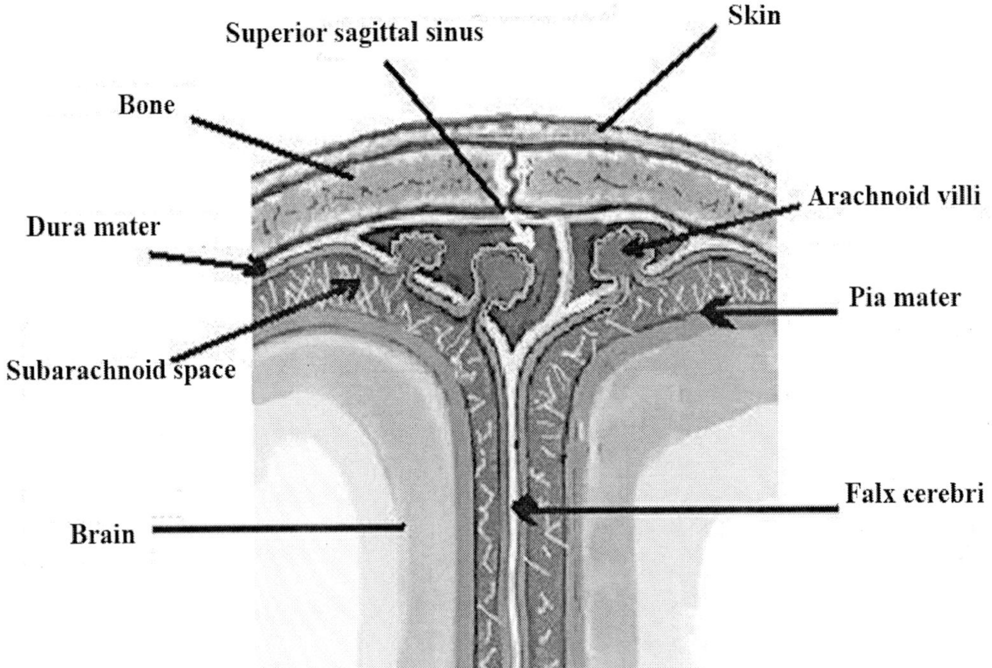

Figure 3. Scheme of the meningeal layers.

2. Nervous Parenchyma

The endocranial content is represented by the nervous tissue, by the endocranial vascular system with a blood content and by the cerebrospinal fluid. [2,3,15]

The volume of the nervous tissue is of approximately 83-88 % of the total endocranial volume, the cerebrospinal fluid is of approximately 100-150 ml, representing 9 % of the endocranial volume, while the blood volume represents approximately 3-7% of the endocranial capacity.

The volume of the endocranial components varies and calculations have established various values for the relation cerebral parenchyma – cerebrospinal fluid – blood: from 80% - 10% - 10% up to 90% - 7% - 3%; the variations are related to individual morphological factors, age, sex, diurnal activity, etc. Thus, after the age of 50 (until approximately 80 years old), the brain volume diminishes by 5-10% (approximately 200 g), while the epicerebral subarachnoid space increases from 6% to 11% of the total endocranial space.

The weight of the encephalon is of approximately 1400 g in the air and of only 50 g in the cerebrospinal fluid. The brain is suspended by the meninx and it floats in the cerebrospinal fluid; CSF allows a slow motion of the intracranial brain during the sudden movements of the head, and it protects the blood vessels and the nervous radices.

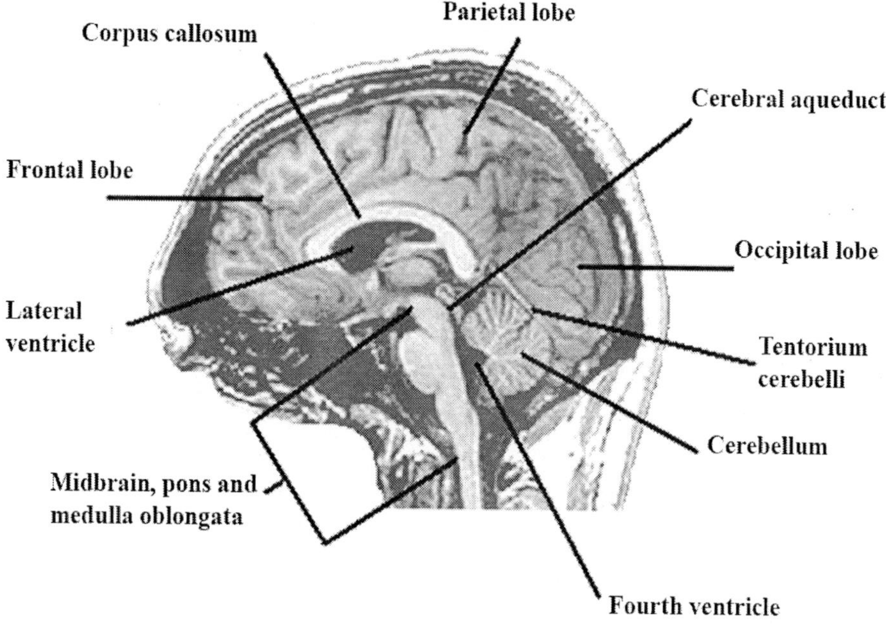

Figure 4. Brain anatomy revealed on a cranial-cerebral MRI, sagittal section

The endocranial nervous tissue is made of neurons and glial cells (central neuroglia): macroglia (astroglia, oligodendroglia, ependymal cells and the choroid epithelial cells) and microglia.

Neuro-glia are smaller than neurons, but more numerous, and they represent approximately half of the nervous tissue. The glial volume is of 700 - 800 cm^3, and the neurons occupy 500 – 700 cm^3 of the endocranial-spinal space.

The extracellular parenchymatous space is occupied by the extracellular fluid or by the interstitial liquid, with a volume of up to 10 % of the total endocranial volume. It may be considered that the neurons and glia cells represent 70 % of the endocranial content, while each of the cerebrospinal fluid, the blood content and the extracellular parenchymatous fluid occupy approximately 10% of the rest of the endocranial space.

Astrocytes represent the most numerous neuroglias. They cover the neurons almost integrally, both the cellular body, and partially the neuronal prolongations; a big part of the neuronal prolongations is covered by oligodendroglia, which forms the myelin sheath. The astrocyte end-feet cover the blood capillaries with small vascular feet; moreover, at the level of the ventricular ependyma, the astrocyte end-feet represent the internal limiting glia, and, from the brain surface, these prolongations get under pia mater, representing the external limiting glia.

The wall of the brain capillaries presents certain characteristics that differentiate it from the other capillaries in the rest of the body: the capillary endothelial cells have junctions of occlusion that do not allow the paracellular passage of substances (among the cells of the capillary wall), representing the brain-blood barrier. The interposition of astrocytes between the blood circulation and the neurons supplements the brain-blood barrier, which is represented by the vascular wall. There are areas that lack a brain-blood barrier: the area postrema, the medial eminence etc.; at this level the cerebral capillaries are fenestrated and a part of the plasma substances may register a paracellular transport into the nervous parenchyma.

The astrocyte end-feet cover the body and the neuronal prolongations, as well as the blood capillaries, and they limit the external cerebral surface and the ventricular walls, thus creating a three-dimensional network that it limits and isolates at peripheries. The nervous cells are included in this network and isolated from any direct contact, except for the one with other neurons; astroglia represents a complex isolating filter for these cells. This three-dimensional neuron-astrocyte-capillary system represents the so-called neuropil.

3. The Ventricular System

The ventricular system includes the anatomic spaces at the encephalon level, which are created due to the modification of the cerebral vesicle lumen during the ontogenetic evolution of the primitive neural tube.[4,8] There are four ventricles that communicate with one another:

- two lateral or telencephalic ventricles,
- the 3rd median ventricle, which continues by
- the aqueduct of *Sylvius* or the cerebral aqueduct, which opens in
- the 4th ventricle, with a median location in the posterior part of the brainstem.

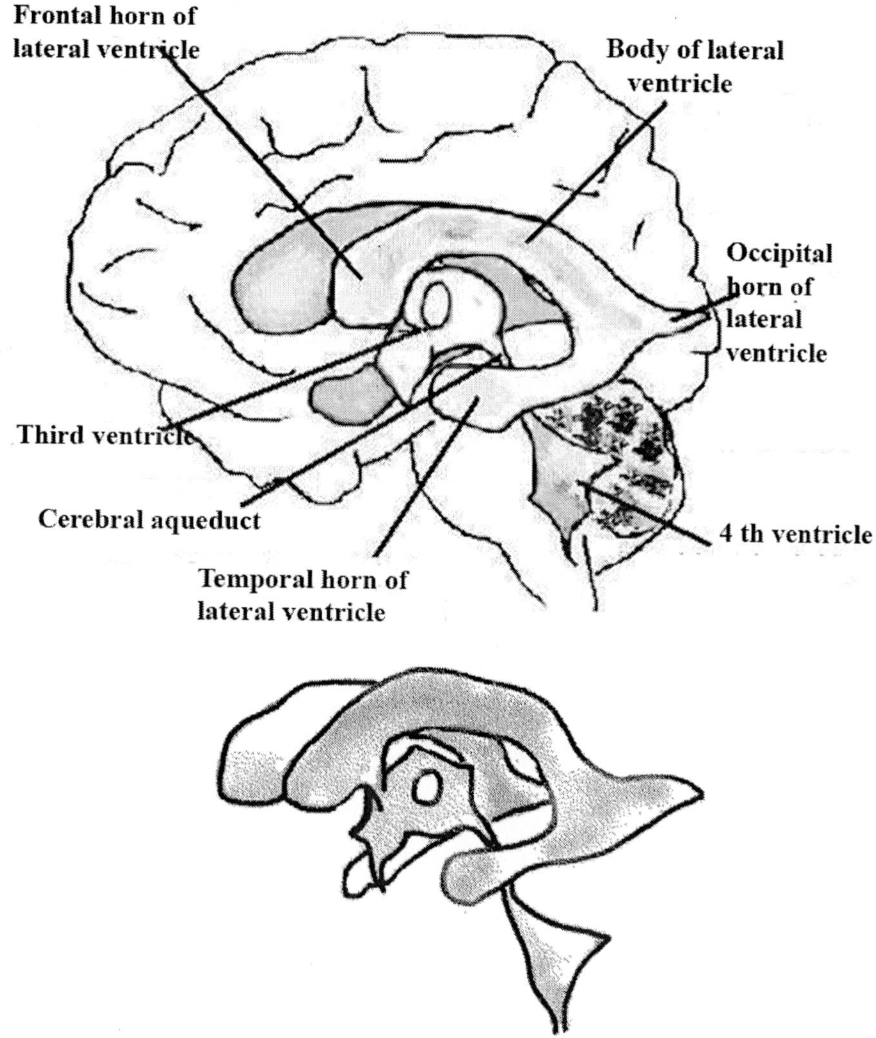

Figure 5. The ventricular system – schematic drawing

Lateral Ventricles

They are represented by the pair and symmetric spaces resulting from the cavities of the telencephalic vesicles. The lateral ventricle resembles a horse shoe in several variants, depending on the form and volume of the encephalon.

The lateral ventricle presents three prolonged portions, which are united in a central area:

- the frontal horn, which has two segments, continuing at the level of the Monro foramen:

  - the frontal cornu, located in the interior of the frontal lobe, at 2.5 cm from the cortical surface

- the body of the lateral ventricle, located in the parietal lobe
- the temporal or sphenoid horn, which is placed in the temporal lobe, having the anterior extremity at up to 1.5 - 2 cm from the temporal pole
- the occipital horn inside the occipital lobe.

- the central part or the ventricular crossway (ventricular trigone or turning point) is the most distended ventricular area, where the ventricular horns meet.

The lateral ventricle includes the caudal nucleus and the posterior part of the thalamus in its concavity.

Usually, the lateral ventricles are not symmetrical and they may present various developments of the horns, especially at the level of the occipital horn, which may be atresic.

The lateral ventricles have the biggest volume in the ventricular system, of approximately 80 %; at young people every lateral ventricle has a volume of 20 - 30 cm^2, which increases in parallel with the age. In an intra-ventricular position and on its concavity, bilaterally, there is the choroid plexus, which has, therefore, the same horse shoe form as the lateral ventricle, and which continues to be with the choroid plexus of the 3rd ventricle at the interventricular foramina (or foramina of Monro).

Third Ventricle

It is odd, situated on the median line, as a narrow cavity with a sagittal orientation, between the diencephalic anatomic formations. The 3rd ventricle communicates with the lateral ventricles by interventricular foramina and it has an inferior continuation by the Sylvian aqueduct. At the level of the 3rd ventricle, there is the superior choroid tissue, which contains the choroid plexuses resulting from the capillaries of the postero-medial choroid artery.

Aqueductus Mesencephali, Aqueduct of Sylvius or the Cerebral Aqueduct

It is a conduct with the approximate length of 2 cm and a caliber of 1.5 mm to 2-3 mm.

Due to its small caliber, it represents a critical area for the ventricular communication, as any intrinsic narrowing (an inflammatory one, etc.) or an extrinsic narrowing (neighbouring compression) eventually blocks the circulation of the cerebrospinal fluid.

Fourth Ventricle

It is an odd, median cavity, with a posterior location from the bridge and the bulb, and an anterior location from the cerebellum. It has an approximately rhombic form, with the big axis in the cranial caudal direction, and it has an inferior continuation by means of the central canal of the spinal cord. The *obex* connects the central canal to the *fourth ventricle.* The posterior infra-cerebellar wall (or the upper limit of the 4th ventricle) includes the tectoria membrane, and it presents an orifice named median aperture of the brain (or foramen of Magendie), which enables the communication between the 4th ventricle and the sub-arachnoid space. At the level of the lateral recesses, the Luschka orifices have been identified, which are not constant, and which also allow the communication with the sub-arachnoid space. The posterior wall in the infra-cerebellar area reveals the inferior choroid tissue, which contains the choroid plexuses of the 4th ventricle, formed by the capillarization of the choroid branches from the postero-inferior cerebellar arteries.

3. Vessels of the Brain and Cerebral Hemodynamics

The encephalon is vascularized by two arterial systems: in the anterior part, the bilateral carotid internal arteries and in the posterior part, the two vertebral arteries; the latter unite at the inferior bridge level and form the basilar trunk. By uniting the branches of the two systems, the carotid and the vertebral ones, the Willis polygon is created at the base of the skull, which may compensate the blocked circulation at the level of a great vessel.[4,8,15] The big cerebral vessels penetrate the subarachnoid space, branch out, participate in the formation of the Willis polygon, which is located in the inter-peduncle cistern, and then enter the nervous parenchyma. Here the arterial and venous vessels are surrounded by the Virchow-Robin peri-vascular spaces, until they become capillaries. In pia-mater thickness, the arterial branches form an arteriolar network; the divided pia-mater constitutes the arteriolar adventitia (the pial peri-arteriolar sheath), and it ends at the beginning of the arteriole capillarization. The cerebral capillaries continue by the venules, which are surrounded by the perivenular spaces, without a pial prolongation.

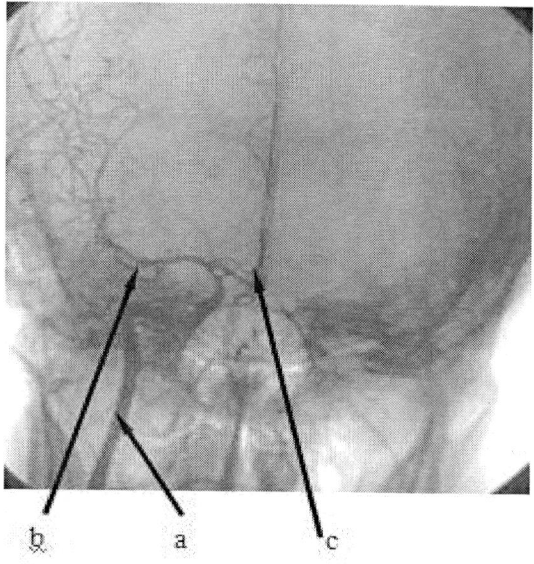

Figure 6. The internal right carotid artery and the intracranial branches, outlined on the right carotid angiography, an antero-posterior image; a = internal right carotid artery, b = middle right cerebral artery. c = anterior right cerebral artery

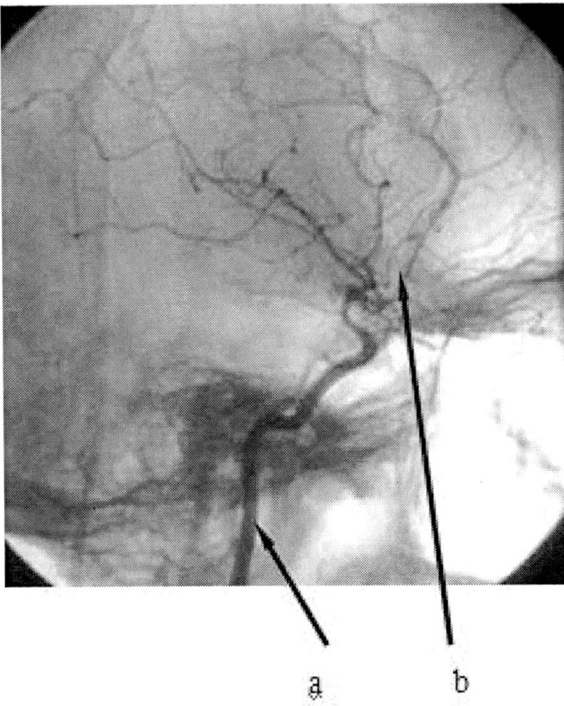

Figure 7. The internal right carotid artery and its branches, outlined on the right carotid angiography, a profile image . a = internal right carotid artery, b =.middle right cerebral artery

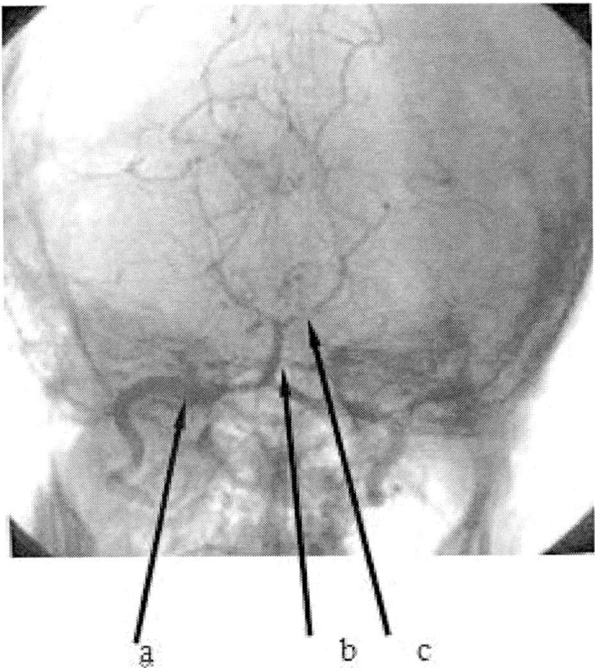

Figure 8. Vertebral arteries - antero-posterior image; , basilar trunk and posterior cerebral arteries, outlined by vertebral angiography, a = right vertebral artery , b = basilar artery ,c = left posterior cerebral artery

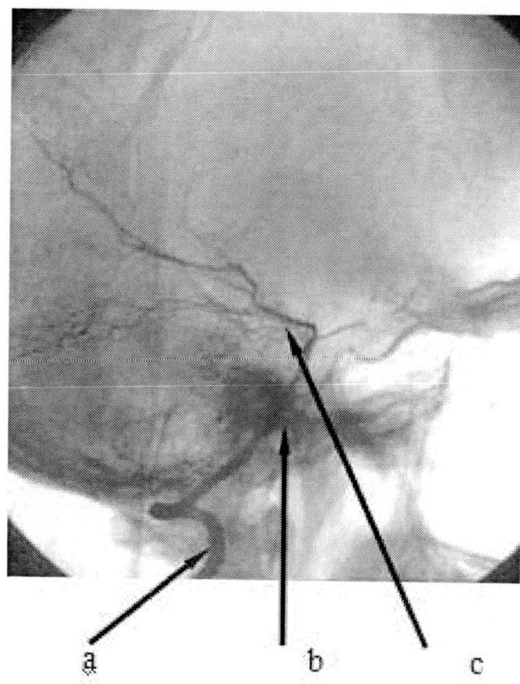

Figure 9. Vertebral angiography – profile image; a = left vertebral artery, b = basilar artery, c = a posterior cerebral artery

The cerebral circulation provides the cerebral parenchyma with a quasi-constant blood flux by means of a complex auto-regulation, which controls the vascular bed. The auto-regulation of the cerebral circulation consists in maintaining a blood flux that is appropriate to the nervous metabolism, and which is not at all or little influenced by the variations of the cerebral perfusion pressure, within certain limits. The factors that establish the circulatory modifications mainly act at the arteriolar-precapillary level by means of several mechanisms that complete one another, and which may gather in order to maintain the cerebral sanguine flux within normal limits. [6,10,14,15]

The auto-regulating mechanisms of the cerebral circulation are considered to be the following ones:

- mechanisms of local and general metabolic regulation;
- myogenous mechanism, by the reaction of the arterial and arteriolar muscular wall to the modifications of the arterial pressure, and
- mechanisms of sympathetic-parasympathetic neurogenic regulation.

1) The local metabolic auto-regulation is achieved by means of the direct connection between the metabolic needs of the nervous parenchyma and the vasomotor modifications brought about by the local metabolism products. Their vasodilating or vasoconstricting action is directly manifested at the level of the arteriolar discontinuous smooth muscles, and at the level of the arteriolar precapillary

sphincters. Modifications occur in the capillarization degree (the number of open capillaries) with a variation of the blood flux according to the local metabolic needs.

2) The general metabolic auto-regulation by the reactivity to the blood gases: carbon dioxide and oxygen. An excessive presence of the CO_2 or the deficit of O_2 leads to a cerebral vasodilatation, while the decrease in the carbon dioxide concentration of the blood that irrigates the brain causes vasoconstriction. The vasomotor action of the blood gas is manifested at the level of the arterioles and of the precapillary sphincters, leading to modifications of the cerebral sanguine flux. The effect of the partial pressure of CO_2 or of O_2 is not correlated to the modifications of the blood pressure.
3) The general metabolic auto-regulation by means of blood viscosity modifications depends on the variations of the plasmatic viscosity and on the values of the hematocrit. The decrease in the blood viscosity, induced by various mechanisms or occurred in particular conditions, generates an increase in the cerebral blood flux, just as the increase in the circulating blood viscosity leads to a decrease in the blood circulation speed. This hemodynamic mechanism is determined by the blood rheological properties, and it observes the Poiseuille law (the draining flow is in inverse proportion to the viscosity of the flowing fluid).
4) The auto-regulation achieved by means of a myogenous mechanism is provided by the reaction of the arterial and arteriolar smooth muscles to the variations of blood pressure. The low blood pressure generates a cerebral vasodilatation in order to maintain the brain perfusion, while the high blood pressure leads to a cerebral vasoconstriction in order to hinder the increase in the capillary pressure, the break of the brain blood barrier and the occurrence of the brain edema. The myogenous auto-regulation is functional between the blood pressure limits of 60 mm Hg to 160 mm Hg, with individual variations; in case of people suffering from high blood pressure, this mechanism may be functional up to higher values than those of the systolic blood pressure, of approximately 180 mm Hg or even up to 200 mm Hg.
5) The neurogenic regulating mechanism of the cerebral circulation depends on the vegetative innervation, secured by the vasomotor plexuses and by the adrenergic and cholinergic receptors of the smooth muscles of the cerebral vessels. The sympathetic innervation is provided by the fibers coming from the superior cervical sympathetic ganglions and by the noradrenergic vascular fibers of a central origin (locus ceruleus), while the cholinergic parasympathetic innervation is caused by the reticulated formation from the medulla oblongata.

These auto-regulating mechanisms function concomitantly or in different sequences based on the metabolic and pressure modifications that are brought about; the local metabolic auto-regulation is the one that permanently secures an appropriate cerebral blood flux, while the other regulating mechanisms become active in situations that may disturb the normal cerebral perfusion.

The cerebral blood flow depends on the cerebral perfusion pressure (CPP), but it is maintained constant by auto-regulation, at values of approximately 50 - 65 mL blood /100 g cerebral tissue /min, with values of 20 mL blood /100g/ min in the white substance up to 70mL blood /100g/ min in the grey substance.

The cerebral blood flow is maintained normal at values of the cerebral perfusion pressure of minimum 70 mm Hg; the blood flow gradually decreases below these values, and a significant decrease in the cerebral blood flow, leading to collapse, occurs for values of the cerebral perfusion below 40 mm Hg.

The oxygen saturation in the jugular venous blood has a normal average of 65% - 75%, but it modifies according to the oxygen extraction rate. The decrease in the cerebral perfusion pressure below 70 mm Hg is rapidly followed by the oxygen saturation decrease in the bulb of the jugular vcin.

The cerebral blood flux is not affected by the moderate variations of the intracranial pressure, but an important ICP increase initially leads to the contraction of the capillaries and the slow-down of the sanguine circulation. The consequence is the secondary CO_2 increase and the decrease in the blood O_2, which generates the increase in the cerebral blood flow with vasodilatation, although the ICP is increased, maintaining the cerebral perfusion pressure.

The intracranial pressure is rapidly influenced by the variations of the cerebral blood volume, which occurs as a factor of instability for ICP. The connection between the cerebral vessels, the dural sinuses and the great vessels of the throat makes it possible for the venous pressure increases, which are induced by the modifications from the level of the thorax or of the throat, to be sent intracranially, being able to influence the intracranial pressure.

5. Brain Blood Barrier

The brain blood barrier (BBB) represents the morpho-functional system with a protecting role, which separates the nervous parenchyma from the blood circulation, in order to secure and control the cerebral homeostasis. It is both an anatomic barrier and a system of physical-chemical and biochemical mechanisms of membrane transport, representing a dynamic interface that regulates the exchanges between the blood circulation and the fluids of the nervous system (the parenchymatous interstitial fluid and the cerebrospinal fluid). The brain blood barrier protects the nervous parenchyma against the harmful substances that may exist in the circulating blood, allowing the supply of the central nervous system with the nourishing substances that are necessary for its appropriate functioning. [6,7,11,14,19]

There are two systems: the actual brain blood barrier and the fluid blood barrier at the level of the choroid plexuses, which is the barrier between the blood and the cerebrospinal fluid.

At the end of the 19th century, Paul Erlich (1885) and many other researchers afterwards, notices that the hydro-soluble coloring substances do not pass from the blood circulation into the brain; in 1900, Lewandowsky uses the term of brain blood barrier ("bluthirnschranke") for the first time.

The profound studies from the second half of the past century underline that the brain blood barrier is anatomically represented by the occlusion junctions (tight junctions) among the endothelial cells of the cerebral capillaries.

Anatomic Structure

The brain blood barrier is made of the endothelial cells of the cerebral capillary wall without fenestrations among them. The cerebral capillary lumen, with its blood content, is limited and completely surrounded by the tightly united endothelial cells, which generates a continuous layer that does not allow any anatomic communication between the capillary lumen and the peri-endothelial structures. The major difference compared to the capillaries existing in the rest of the body consists in the absence of the fenestrations that may allow the endothelial paracellular passage (through the cells of the capillary wall). The occlusion junctions or "zonulae occludens", also named the tight or impermeable cell junctions, result from the anastomosis of the junction proteins that are present in the plasmatic membranes of the neighbouring endothelial cells, and they hinder the motion of molecules and ions from the capillary lumen. They maintain the membrane stability of the capillary endothelial cells and allow the cerebral capillary endothelium to behave as a barrier with selective permeability. [1,5,12,13,16]

The endothelial cells have their extra-luminal pole on a thin basal membrane; on this basal membrane where prolongations are sent, there are pericytes, which surround up to 30 % of the cerebral capillary circumference. The basal membrane is presented as a protein layer that surrounds the blood capillary, separates the adjacent tissues (the capillary endothelium is separated from the astrocyte end-feet), it is the mechanical support for the fixation of cells, allows the migration of pericytes, and it is a barrier for the passage of macro-molecules.

At the level of the peripheral capillaries, pericytes play the part of contractile cells, but, at the level of the cerebral micro-circulation, pericytes act in the mechanisms of endothelial cellular proliferation by inhibiting the cellular development. The absence of pericytes leads to an abnormal cerebral vascular morphogenesis.

The cerebral capillaries are surrounded by the the astrocyte end-feet, which are presented in contact with the basal membrane of the cerebral capillary. The peri-capillary astrocyte end-feet interact with the cerebral capillary endothelium and they stimulate the creation of the occlusion junctions at the level of the endothelial cells, providing the selective permeability properties that maintain the barrier function of the capillary endothelium.

Among the astrocyte end-feet, which are applied on the basal membrane of the cerebral capillary, there are:

- anchoring junctions ("zonulae adherens"), which secure the intracellular adhesion to the extracellular matrix and to the endothelial basal membrane, and
- communicating junctions (permeable, "gap junctions"), structures with a dynamic character, permeable in relation to pH, ionic concentration, electric potential, etc.

These characteristics of the astrocyte end-feet that surround the cerebral capillaries show that they do not take part in the physical barrier that separates the blood circulation from the cerebral parenchyma, as these junctions are permeable (paracellular diffusion).

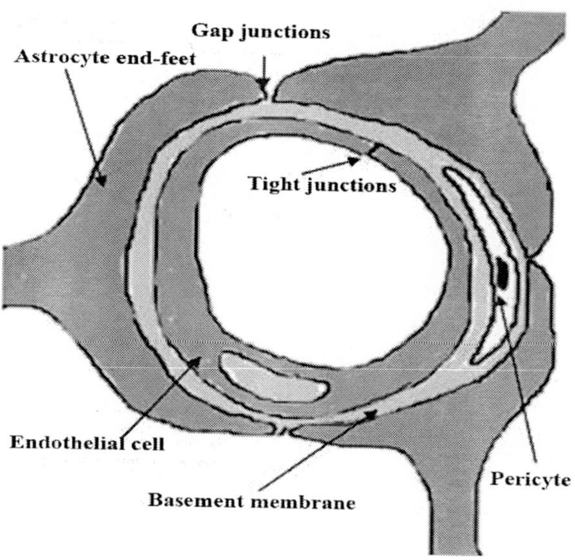

Figure 10. Scheme of the brain blood barrier .

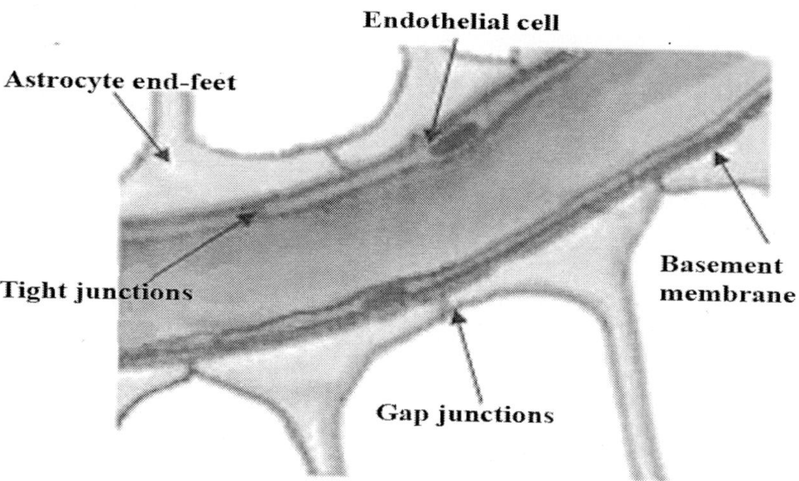

Figure 11. Scheme of the cerebral capillary – brain blood barrier .

Physiology

The brain blood barrier is present at birth, but it is incompletely developed at the premature new-born baby or even at the normal new-born baby; its development continues after birth too. This means that in the case of a new-born baby the central nervous system is sensitive to the toxins that overcome the brain-blood barrier.

The central nervous system includes several areas that lack the brain-blood barrier: these are the so-called circumventricular organs, which are nervous structures around the 3rd and the 4th ventricles. These structures include: the pineal gland, the median eminence, the neurohypophysis, the subfornical organ, the area postrema, the sub-commissural organ, and the organum vasculosum of the terminal lamina.

The choroid plexuses constitute the hemato-fluid barrier, they present the fenestrated and permeable endothelium of the blood capillaries, and the cerebrospinal fluid is produced at this level.

Recent studies show that, beside the mechanical role of tissue separation and of a selective barrier for macro-molecules, the capillary basal membrane acts as the second component of the brain-blood barrier, as a filter, by blocking certain simple substances that have passed by the capillary endothelium. From a structural point of view, the basal membrane is presented as a network made of laminins, fibronectins, tenascins, collagen and proteoglycans, and it has been compared to a "cobweb" where simple substances or viral particles are kept in pathological situations. Experiments have been performed with nano-particles of iron oxide, which manage to pass the capillary endothelium, surpassing the basal membrane only by means of an association with certain substances (crystallized nanoparticles of iron oxide, covered with dextran, generating the preparation ferumoxtran-10, which may be used in the exploration of the cerebral IMR). The mechanisms, by means of which the substances that have passed the capillary endothelium are blocked at the level of the basal membrane, are yet uncertain; they seem to function as a filter by the combination between the network anatomic structure and an electrically loaded barrier.

The functioning of the brain blood barrier is secured by the selective membrane transport mechanisms, based on which exchanges are regulated between the blood circulation and the fluid of the nervous system.[5,9,13,18]

The transport through the cerebral capillary endothelium is fulfilled by means of several mechanisms:

- the simple diffusion of ions and small molecules, caused by their concentration or electrochemical gradient: O_2, CO_2, NO, H^+, Na^+, Cl^-, K^+, ethanol, nicotine, etc. The crossing of the double-membrane lipid layer is easier for liposoluble substances that have a bigger permeability constant. Molecules must cross the luminal membrane of the capillary endothelial cell, then they move through the cytoplasm of the endothelial cell towards the basal pole, and then the crossing of the basal membrane of the capillary endothelial cell takes place. The next step is the crossing of the basal membrane with a passage into the astrocyte end-feet or the passage through the permeable junctions between the astrocyte feet in the inter-glial interstitial matrix and the entrance in the astrocyte.
- the simple diffusion by means of the "water channels", facilitated by aquaporins ("the water channel protein" in the double lipid membrane layer), resulting from the action of the concentration difference or / and the hydrostatic pressure gradient.
- the facilitated diffusion, which also depends on the concentration gradient, is a passive transport, mediated by the membrane proteins and characterized by the specificity of the transported molecule. Due to the facilitated diffusion, the brain blood barrier is crossed by glucose, hexosamines, amino-acids, nucleosides, glutathione, small peptides, etc.

- active transport, which is mediated by specific proteins. The transporting molecule has an ATPase function, and thus the active transport of the ions of Na^+, K^+, Ca^{2+} is produced regardless of their concentration gradients and electrochemically.
  There are three classes of proteins that may perform the active transport:
  a) the class of ATP-ases-P, which are trans-membrane proteins, and the transport is performed by dividing the ATP into ADP and inorganic phosphor (P), with the following representatives: Na^+- K^+- ATP- ase (Na^+- K^+ pump) and Ca^{2+}- ATP- ase (Ca^{2+}pump).
  b) the class of hydrogen - ATP-ases and
  c) the class of proton- ATP-ases. The transport of the same substance may be achieved at different moments and in several ways: simple diffusion or active transport depending on the homeostasic needs

- the vesicle-mediated transport: pinocytosis, endocytosis and transcytosis.

  a. The pinocytosis is non-specific, it depends on temperature and it is non-competitive (Simionescu, 1987); the pinocytosis enables the penetration of solution molecules into the cell. The pinocytosis is produced in a reduced degree at the level of the cerebral capillary circulation (Partridge, 1995).
  b. The endocytosis is mediated by membrane receptors and it is specific. It consists in recognizing and connecting macromolecules to the membrane receptors, after which the macromolecule-receptor complex enters the cell with no extra-cellular fluid. The macromolecule-receptor complex manifests an invagination; a vesicle is formed, which is internalized, and then becomes an endosome. At the membrane level, the endothelial cells of the cerebral

     capillaries contain receptors for hormones, growing factors, enzymes and plasmatic proteins. Receptors for transferrins (Fishman, 1987), insulin (Duffy and Partridge, 1987), leptins (Banks, 1996) etc. have been identified.
  c. Transcytosis is a trans-cellular specific transport of macromolecules and it requires the vesicles containing the macromolecule-receptor complex to cross the cellular space until they reach the basal region of the endothelial cell, where they cross the cellular membrane and the macromolecule that is dissociated by the receptor.

The passive transport is simply required by the difference of concentration between fluids in contact. The active and vesicle-mediated transport is generated by the nervous parenchyma due to a decrease in the concentration of the necessary substances and an increase in the quantities of the substances that must be eliminated.

Several layers are crossed by the necessary substances in order to reach the neuron:

- the wall of the cerebral capillary by passive and active transport mechanisms:
  - the luminal membrane of the endothelial cell
  - the basal membrane of the endothelial cell
- the basement membrane, sometimes through the pericytes, the passage is a filtration,

- the astrocyte level :
  - the interglial interstitial space
  - the pericapillary astrocyte end-feet, with inter-astrocyte communicating junctions, the passage of substances is also a filtration
  - the cellular body of the astrocyte until the peri-neuronal astrocyte end-feet are reached
- the neuronal membrane.

The surface of the cerebral capillaries is of approximately 100 cm^2 / g up to 180 cm^2 / g of nervous tissue, the volume of the capillaries in the nervous parenchyma represents approximately 1 % of the cerebral volume, while the volume of the endothelial cells of the cerebral capillaries represents approximately 0.1 % of the cerebral volume.

The endothelial cells and the basal membranes of the cerebral capillaries are thinner than those at the level of the peripheral capillaries, having a thickness that is about 1/3 smaller, which allows an easier functioning of the transport mechanisms. The distance between the cerebral blood capillaries is of approximately 40 μm and this very small distance allows the fluid from the interstitial space (the interglial space) to have a quasi-constant composition by means of an extremely fast equilibration.

Modifications of the Brain Blood Barrier

The parenchymatous interstitial fluid has the same composition as the cerebrospinal fluid, both of them resulting from the functioning of the two barriers that separate the blood circulation from the nervous parenchyma, securing the same result in order to control the cerebral homeostasis. The mechanisms, based on which the macromolecule passage is achieved by the brain-blood barrier, have been intensely studied during the past few years in view of various therapeutic applications or for cerebral exploration.

The capacity of various substances to cross the brain blood barrier depends on several factors at the level of the cerebral capillary:

- inter-compartmental concentration,
- molecule size,
- conformation and flexibility of macromolecules,
- permeability and lipo-solubility degree,
- types of membrane receptors, etc.,

and at the level of the cerebral circulation:

- the surface of the available cerebral capillaries,
- the cerebral blood flux,
- the type of plasmatic proteins,
- the existence of certain pathological situations, etc.

Numerous illnesses of the central nervous system are based on the mechanism that increases the permeability of the brain blood barrier for fluids or various substances, with different anatomic-clinical aspects: brain edema, inflammation, radioactive exposure, cerebral ischemia and reperfusion, intracranial hypertension, etc.

Various factors may cause modifications of the brain-blood barrier:

- opening of the occlusion junctions :
  - due to the action of certain hyperosmolary substances
  - pH modification
  - the inflammatory action of certain substances such as bradykinin, histamine etc.

  or
  - the complex mechanisms that occur in the cerebral post-ischemic reperfusion
- the absence of the occlusion junctions of the neo-formation sanguine capillaries in cerebral glial tumors as the neoplasic astrocytes no longer induce the occurrence of this type of endothelial junction; the neo-formation capillaries are numerous, they are fenestrated, with communication junctions and with numerous vesicles of pinocytosis
- the opening of more membrane passage channels
  - under the action of certain drugs, such as the three-cyclic anti-depressives
  - in an acute episode of high blood pressure– water channels
- the emphasis on the vesicle mediated transport in numerous pathological conditions:
  - cerebral ischemia
  - comitial crises
  - traumatic brain injury
  - meningitis etc.
- modification of the membrane physical properties by
  - ethanol,
  - various liposoluble solvents: propanol, buthanol
- modifications of the normal transport conditions occurred in certain illnesses :
  - diabetes mellitus
  - thiamine insufficiency in Korsakoff syndrome
  - Alzheimer disease, etc.

The homeostasis of the nervous parenchyma is secured by the appropriate functioning of the brain-blood barrier, which occupies a central position in the occurrence and development of the central nervous system pathology by regulating the exchanges with the sanguine circulation.

6. The Cerebrospinal Fluid

The cerebrospinal fluid (CSF) is the biological fluid that is present in the cerebral ventricular system, in the medullar ependymal channel, as well as in the subarachnoid spaces. Most of it is produced at the level of the ventricular choroid plexuses, and its resorption is achieved mainly by means of the arachnoid vilosities in the cranial venous sinuses. The total volume of the cerebrospinal fluid is of approximately 150 mL at an adult, of which approximately 25 - 30 mL in the ventricular system, other 30 mL in the spinal subarachnoid space, while the rest of the cerebrospinal fluid is included in the subarachnoid cranial space and in the basal cisterns. The medullar ependymal channel is sometimes in a collapse, with no cerebrospinal fluid or with a very small quantity of cerebrospinal fluid. [2,4,8,19]

The cerebrospinal fluid has several functions:

- it has a nourishing role, taking part in metabolic exchanges and in providing the biochemical stability of the nervous parenchyma,
- it plays a part in the neuro-endocrine integrity of the levels of the central nervous system by means of the hormonal circulation,
- it has a hydrostatic role, due to the force of Archimedes lift, securing the floatability of the brain; the weight of the brain in the cerebrospinal fluid is of approximately 50 grams,
- it has a mechanical protection role, by the absorption of shocks during head motions,
- it plays a part in maintaining the temperature of the central nervous system.

Production of the Cerebrospinal Fluid

Approximately 60 % - 70 % of the cerebrospinal fluid is elaborated by the choroid plexuses from the cerebral ventricles. The choroid plexuses separate the blood circulation from the cerebrospinal fluid, representing the fluid blood barrier of the central nervous system. The choroid plexuses are located in the lateral ventricles, in the 3rd and 4th ventricles.

The ventricular system is formed after the closing, curving and development of the neural tube, and it communicates with the sub-arachnoid space by the Luschka and Magendie foramens; the ventricular system and the subarachnoid space are completely developed at birth, and they contain cerebrospinal fluid. [4,7,10,17]

The choroid plexuses are included in the prolongations of the pia mater, which register an intra-ventricular penetration:

- at the level of the lateral ventricle, pia mater is engaged by the choroid sulcus from the inner side of the temporal lobe, covering the choroid artery vessels. The choroid arterial branches, which are capillarized, forming the choroid plexuses at this level, come from the previous choroid artery, as a branch of the internal choroid artery, and from the posterior-lateral choroid artery, as a branch of the posterior cerebral artery. The choroid plexuses from the lateral ventricles have a surface of approximately 40 cm^2 and they produce the biggest quantity of cerebrospinal fluid.
- at the level of the 3rd ventricle, pia mater forms the tela chorioidea of the third ventricle, which includes the choroid plexuses formed by the capillarization of the posterior-medial choroid artery branches, which come from the posterior cerebral arteries. The choroid plexuses of the 3rd ventricle continue by the choroid plexuses of the lateral ventricles.

- at the level of the 4th ventricle, pia mater forms the tela chorioidea of the fourth ventricle, which includes the choroid plexuses reached by the choroid branches from the posterior-inferior cerebellar arteries, branches of the vertebral artery. At the level of the lateral recesses of the 4th ventricle, there are the Luschka orifices (but they may be absent quite often), and the choroid plexuses of the 4th ventricle penetrate the sub-arachnoid space by means of these orifices.

The choroid plexuses are formed by the capillarization of the choroid arteries; the capillaries are surrounded by a conjunctive tissue and they come in contact with the ependymal epithelium by means of the basement membrane. The capillaries of the choroid plexuses are different from the rest of the cerebral capillaries because they have fenestrations by which the substances pass from the capillary lumen towards the ependymal epithelium. The ependymal cells that cover the choroid capillaries present circumferential occlusion junctions that join them together and allow a selective permeability. The ependymal cells of the choroid plexuses have a voluminous nucleus, they have numerous cellular organelles (mitochondrias, lyso-somes, pinocytary vesicles) and an abundant cytoplasm with a rich enzymatic content, which underlines an intense metabolic activity for the elaboration of the cerebrospinal fluid.

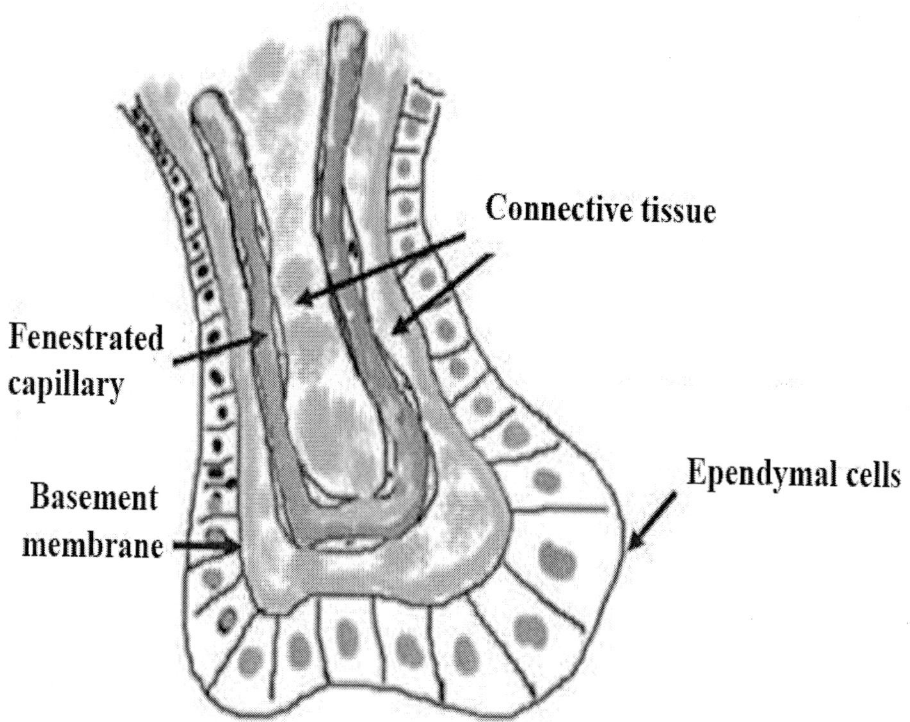

Figure 12. Structure of the choroid plexuses.

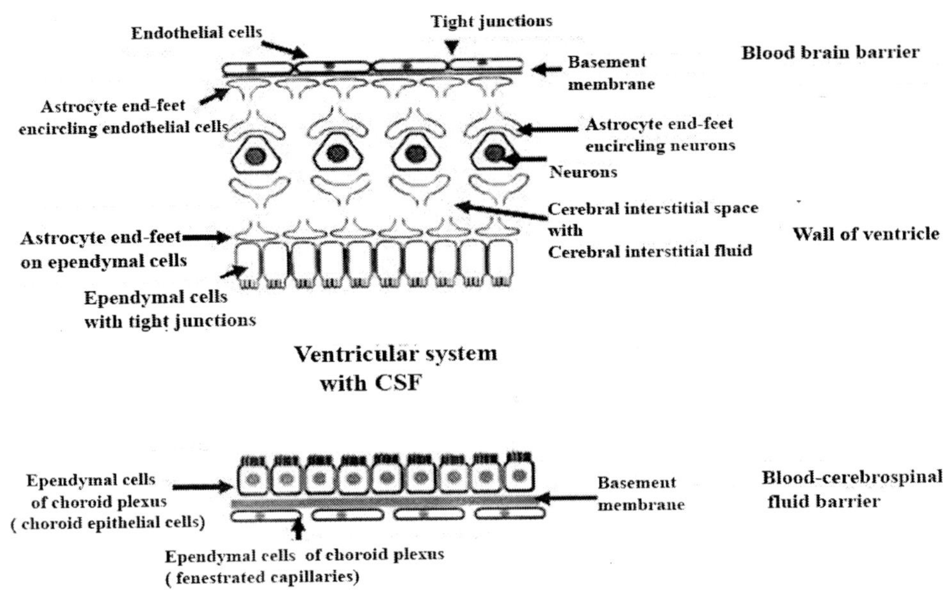

Figure 13. Brain-blood barrier, the ventricular wall and the choroid plexus.

The composition of the cerebrospinal fluid is identical with the one of the nervous parenchymatous interstitial fluid, which means that the exchanges between the blood circulation and the fluids of the nervous system are based on the same transport membrane mechanisms.

The production of the cerebrospinal fluid is accomplished in two stages: the passage through the wall of the capillaries into the choroid plexus and the trans-ependymal passage.

At the level of the choroid plexuses, there is, at first, an ultra-filtration process of the blood plasma from the fenestrated choroid capillaries, and then there is an intra-ventricular selective transfer by means of an active transport at the level of the choroid ependymal cell.

At the level of the basement membrane at of the choroid ependymal cell, the transport is achieved by means of several mechanisms with different shares: simple diffusion, simple diffusion by “water channels”, facilitated by aquaporins, facilitated diffusion, active transport and vesicle mediated transport.

The transport of the ions of sodium, chlorine, etc. is an active transport that is mediated by Na+/K+-ATPase (Na+/K+ pump), which is mostly dependent on the carbonic anhydrase. The intra-ventricular passage of water seems to be a mechanism of simple diffusion, which is mediated by aquaporins, as a reply to the passage of the sodium ions. The passage of the other substances from the blood plasma into the cerebrospinal fluid is performed by the transfer mechanisms presented above.

The cerebrospinal fluid has the same components as the blood plasma, but their concentration is different; the mechanisms that elaborates the cerebrospinal fluid is a mechanism of ultra-filtration at the level of the choroid capillary endothelium and a mechanism of selective transportation at the level of the ependymal cells. [6,17]

Table 2. The comparative composition of the cerebrospinal fluid and of the blood serum

Substance	Cerebrospinal fluid	Blood serum
Sodium (mEq / L)	140	140
Potassium (mEq / L)	2.9	4.6
Chlorine (mEq / L)	124	101
Bicarbonate (mEq / L)	21	23
Glucoses (mg / 100 mL)	60	90
Proteins (mg / 100 mL)	20 – 30	7000
pH	7.30	7.4
Osmolarity (mOsm/L)	289	289

The cerebrospinal fluid is not a secretion since it is not a product elaborated by the ependymal cells, but it results from the selective permeability provided by the coupling of the endothelial filtration with the active ependymal transport.

The mechanisms that elaborate the cerebrospinal fluid at the level of the choroid plexuses – passage through filtration, followed by an active ependymal cellular transport – are the same mechanisms that generate the interstitial fluid at the level of the brain blood barrier – active endothelial cellular transport, followed by a passage through filtration at the level of the astrocyte end-feet.

The generation of the cerebrospinal fluid depends on the pressure of the cerebral perfusion, and the decrease in the perfusion pressure at the level of the choroid vessels below 50 mm Hg leads to the a poorer filtration of the choroid capillary filtration and a decrease in the elaboration of the cerebrospinal fluid.

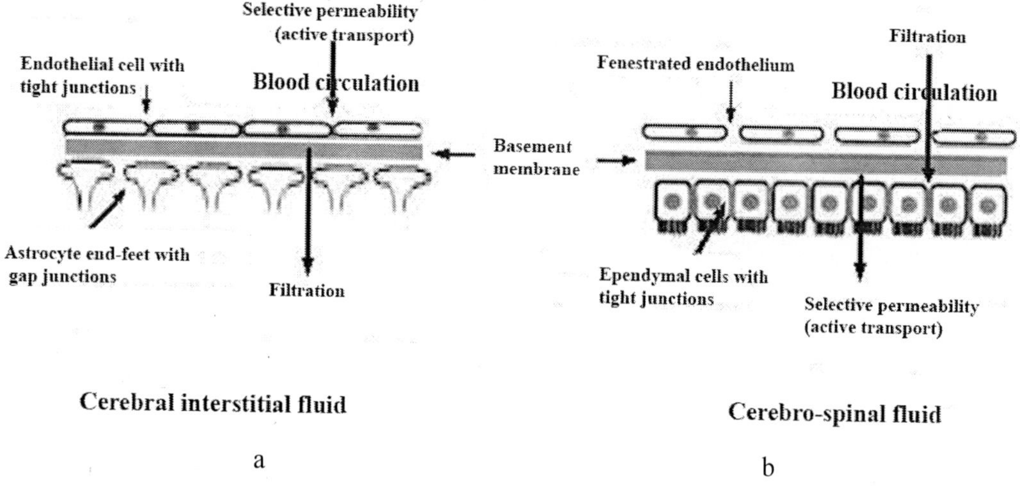

Figure 14. Comparative presentation of the brain blood barrier (a) and of the blood-cerebrospinal fluid barrier, as well as of the transport mechanisms: identical filtration and selective permeability, but in a reversed order .

The volume of the cerebrospinal fluid is considered to be equal to the volume of the extracellular fluid in the parenchymatous interstitial space.

The cerebrospinal fluid and the parenchymatous interstitial fluid are elaborated by the same mechanisms, but in a reversed order due to the anatomic particularities regarding each type of barrier.

The brain blood barrier corresponds to a big number of capillaries, which secure a very large exchange area (the surface of the cerebral capillaries is of 100 - 180 cm^2 / g cerebral tissue). This allows the selective permeability of the barrier to perform the passage by means of an active transport as a first step, which is energy-consuming and slower, but which promptly meets the local glial-neuronal needs. The next step is a much faster passage through the endothelial basement membrane and through the communication junctions of the astrocyte end-feet as a filtration phenomenon. The blood-cerebrospinal fluid barrier has a very small exchange area compared to the brain blood barrier and the first step is the rapid filtration by the fenestrated capillary endothelium, followed by the mechanisms of active transport at the level of the ependymal cells.

The two barriers have the same functioning mechanisms and the result is the same: the two resulting fluids have the same composition and they are produced in equivalent quantities.

The parenchymatous interstitial fluid has the major role of providing the nervous parenchyma with the necessary substances, while the cerebrospinal fluid has a more important role in removing the catabolites resulting from the nervous metabolism.

The rest of 30 - 40 % of the cerebrospinal fluid comes from the level of the extra-choroid sources. These sources are represented by the pia mater capillaries and by the trans-ependymal exchanges at the level of the ventricular walls. The ependymal basement membrane is absent at the level of the ventricular wall, and there are communicating junctions between the ependymal cells, which allows the permanent passage of the interstitial fluid in the ventricular system and the completion of the cerebrospinal fluid.

The cerebrospinal fluid is produced at an approximate rhythm of 0.20 – 0.70 mL / min, with an average of 0.35 mL/ min, which is the equivalent of 12 - 40 mL per hour, with an average of 21 mL per hour or about 600 - 700 mL per day; therefore, during one day, the quantity of cerebrospinal fluid is replaced at least three times.

The normal quantity of cerebrospinal fluid is of 40 - 50 mL at infants and it increases progressively in parallel to the body development, reaching the level of 150 mL at adults.

The Circulation of the Cerebrospinal Fluid

The circulation of the cerebrospinal fluid starts from the ventricular system towards the subarachnoid space, through Magendie foramen at the level of the 4th ventricular. The cerebrospinal fluid from the lateral ventricles passes into the 3rd ventricle by Monro orifices, then by the Sylvian aqueduct, arriving in the 4th ventricle. The cerebrospinal fluid passes from the 4th ventricle into the magna cistern through Magendie foramen, and, from this point, it travels throughout the subarachnoid space. There is another classical description of the passage of the cerebrospinal fluid from the 4th ventricle into the bridge cistern by Lushka's foramens, but the modern anatomy data have not established the constant behaviour of these orifices.

The cerebrospinal fluid follows three directions from the magna cistern:

- towards the cerebellum subarachnoid system
- towards prepontine, interpeduncular and suprasellar basal cisterns
- towards the spinal subarachnoid space.

The cerebrospinal fluid travels from the basal cisterns towards the basal and then lateral faces of the cerebral hemispheres, and towards the internal sides of the cerebral hemispheres. At the level of the spinal canal, the cerebrospinal fluid descends on the posterior side of the spinal cord, it touches the pouch of the dural sac, and then climbs the anterior side of the cord until it reaches the basal cisterns. The fluid circulation is a pulsatile one and the motion of the cerebrospinal fluid takes place in two stages, in relation to the cardiac activity: a systolic phase with a faster movement and a diastolic phase with a slower movement. These two phases have an equal duration in the lateral ventricles, but, the further the liquid flow gets from the generating source, the duration of the phase with the fast systolic movement decreases, so that, at the level of the sub-arachnoid phase, the slow motion phase becomes the dominant one, and, at the level of the dural sac pouch, only a constant slow liquid flow may be noticed.

The circulation of the cerebrospinal fluid is guided by the pressure difference of the cerebrospinal fluid at the moment of elaboration, as well as by the pressure existing at the resorption place. Moreover, it depends on the movements of the ependymal cilia, on the intracranial arterial pulsations, on respiration, on the modification of the head position, and it is influenced by physical efforts and by any causes that lead to an intracranial pressure.

Concomitantly to this circulation on the anatomic paths occupied by the cerebrospinal fluid, there are permanent fluid exchanges between the parenchymatous extracellular fluid and the cerebrospinal fluid, at the trans-ependymal level and at the pial trans-cerebral one, and these fluid exchanges represent a slow transversal circulation.

Resorption of the Cerebrospinal Fluid

The resorption of the cerebrospinal fluid is fulfilled at the level of the dural venous sinuses by means of the arachnoid granulations. The arachnoid granulations are arachnoid prolongations into the thickness of the dura mater and of the venous sinuses, which hypertrophy by the age, they may leave prints on the internal skull-cap and they have been named corpuscles or Pacchioni's granulations.

The passage of the cerebrospinal fluid from the subarachnoid space into the venous sinuses is achieved by means of a unidirectional valvular mechanism and by a vesicle-mediated trans-cellular transport. The arachnoid granulations secure the resorption of the cerebrospinal fluid up to 60 - 80 % of its total volume.

The resorption of the cerebrospinal fluid is also achieved at other levels:

- the arachnoid granulations are also present at the arachnoid sheaths of the spinal nerves, and, at this level, the cerebrospinal fluid passes into the peri-radicular veins,
- a lymphatic resorption: by means of the leptomeningeal sheaths of the cranial and spinal nerves until it reaches the exit of the cranial-spinal space where there are lymphatic vessels
- the trans-ependymal path, at the level of the ventricular walls: the cerebrospinal fluid crosses the ventricular ependyma, opposite to the normal circuit, it passes into the cerebral parenchyma and it is drained in the cerebral capillaries. The mechanism is partially efficient in hydrocephalus and it is a fundamental mechanism in the case of idiopathic intracranial hypertension.
- the direct resorption from the subarachnoid space on the path of the cortical capillaries.

The resorption of the cerebrospinal fluid depends directly on the pressure difference between the subarachnoid space and the venous blood in the superior sagittal sinus.

Usually, the pressure gradient is of 3 - 4 mm Hg, but the pressure from the superior sagittal sinus is frequently negative. There is a pressure difference named "critical opening pressure", with an approximate value of 5 mm Hg, after which the resorption of the cerebrospinal fluid is constant, the absorption rate depending only on the pressure values of the cerebrospinal fluid at the level of the arachnoid granulations.

The resorption rate of the cerebrospinal fluid may be calculated based on the pressure gradient between the two compartments and on the flowing resistance at the level of the arachnoid villi.

The conductance is the reverse of the flow resistance and, in the normal conditions of a man's cerebrospinal fluid circulation, it has the value of 0.075 mL / min / mm Hg (or 0.056 mL / min / cm H_2O).

Therefore

Resorption rate = Pressure gradient (CSF – Venous sinus) / Flowing resistance

or

Resorption rate = Pressure gradient (cerebrospinal fluid – Venous sinus) x Conductance

and, for the critical opening pressure, at which a constant resorption of the cerebrospinal fluid is secured, the resorption rate is of 0.35 mL / minute.

In the conditions of a constant cerebral sanguine flux, due to the maintenance of the difference between the blood pressure and the intracranial pressure, there is equilibrium between the production rate of the cerebrospinal fluid and its resorption rate, and thus the volume of the cerebrospinal fluid remains quasi-constant.

7. Dynamics of Intracranial Fluids

The intracranial hydrodynamic processes consist in the development of the circulation and of the intracranial fluid exchanges: blood, parenchymatous interstitial fluid and the cerebrospinal fluid.

The cerebral parenchyma includes these fluids, which may be free or mediated by specific structures (blood vessels), and it is included in the cerebrospinal fluid, on the particular conditions of the limited endocranial volume.

The intracranial arterial vascularization is secured by the internal carotid arteries in a bilateral anterior position, and by the two vertebral arteries in a posterior position. The great cerebral vessels penetrate the subarachnoid space, they form the Willis polygon at the skull base in the inter-peduncular cistern, and then they ramify and enter the nervous parenchyma. The blood vessels are surrounded by Virchow-Robin perivascular spaces here, until they turn into capillaries. The cerebral capillaries continue by venules, surrounded by the perivenular spaces, and then they turn into big veins that flow into the venous sinuses of dura mater. The venous blood from all the intracranial dural sinuses is drained in the lateral sinuses, which continue by the internal jugular veins at the exit from the skull. [6, 7,10,15]

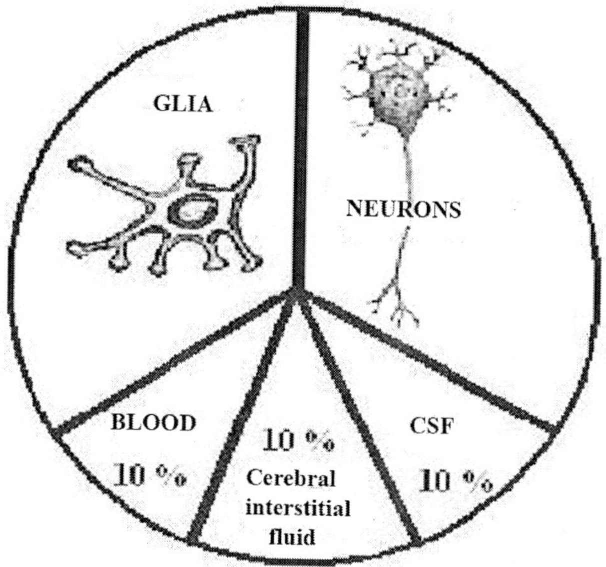

Figure 15. Distribution of the intracranial volumes: 2/3 cerebral parenchyma, consisting of equal shares of neurons and glia, and 1/3 extracellular intracranial fluids.

The cerebral capillaries form two similar structural systems, which have analogous functions based on the same mechanisms of membrane transfer:

- the brain-blood barrier, whose functioning leads to the elaboration of the parenchymatous interstitial fluid, which fulfills the metabolic exchanges that are necessary for an appropriate functioning of the nervous parenchyma, and
- the blood-cerebrospinal fluid barrier at the level of the choroid plexuses, where the cerebrospinal fluid is generated, a fluid that also has metabolic functions, but mechanical protection functions, too.

After its production, the interstitial fluid participates in the glial-neuronal metabolic exchanges, and then it turns to the opposite direction into the sanguine capillaries and into the circulating sanguine flux. Moreover, at the level of the ventricular wall, there is a trans-ependymal passage of the parenchymatous interstitial fluid into the ventricular system, generating permanent exchanges with the cerebrospinal fluid.

The cerebrospinal fluid elaborated in the lateral ventricles passes into the 3rd ventricle and then, by means of the Sylvian aqueduct, it arrives in the 4th ventricle; from this point, it passes into the magna cistern by Magendie's foramen, and it circulates in the sub-arachnoid space. The cerebrospinal fluid is resorbed at the level of the dural venous sinuses by means of the arachnoid granulations.

The two fluids that are elaborated by the functioning of the two types of capillary barriers are identical, and they are produced in the same quantity, each of them representing approximately 10% of the intracranial volume. Moreover, the blood volume circulating at a given moment represents approximately 10% of the total endocranial volume too.

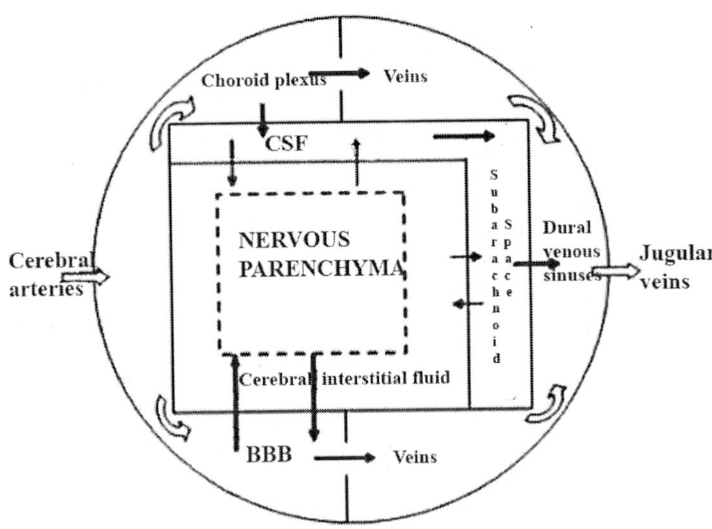

Figure 16. Scheme of the intracranial fluids dynamics .

According to the relation regarding the cranial-cerebral constancy of volumes, postulated by Monro and Kellie: the intradural endocranial volume is constant and its content is incompressible. This means, first of all, that the blood volume with intracranial penetration must be equal to the one that leaves the skull at the same moment, on the condition that the other intracranial components do not modify their volumes. The volumes of the three intracranial fluids are approximately equal, and the exchanges among them are equivalent in order to maintain the constancy of the total endocranial volume on normal pressure conditions.

As far as the fluid distribution is concerned, the intracranial space may be divided in several compartments or sectors:

- the arterial sector, which includes big arteries to arterioles,
- the parenchymatous capillary sector, which corresponds to the brain-blood barrier, and which is the source that generates the creation of the parenchymatous interstitial fluid
- the capillary sector of the choroid plexuses corresponds to the blood-cerebrospinal fluid barrier and it is the place where the cerebrospinal fluid is formed
- the venous sector, which includes the veins, from venules to big veins.
- the sector of the venous sinuses, where the venous blood brought by the big cerebral veins is drained.

  These five compartments represent the intracranial blood circulation.
- the sector of the parenchymatous interstitial fluid, which corresponds to the intercellular space. The interstitial fluid is in a permanent and rapid circulation, as there are two circuits:

  a. the production and resorption circuit at the level of the parenchymatous blood capillary, a rapid circuit, and
  b. the transfer circuit towards the cerebrospinal fluid, a slower one.
- the sector of the cerebrospinal fluid, which includes the ventricular system and the sub- arachnoid space. The circulation of the cerebrospinal fluid is also permanently, and it includes
  a. the fluid circulation through the pre-formed anatomic spaces, from production to resorption
  b. the mutual transfer circuit with the interstitial fluid

- the parenchymatous sector, which includes the neurons and the glial cells, mainly the astrocytes and the oligodendrocytes. The nervous parenchyma includes the interstitial fluid in the intercellular space and the cerebrospinal fluid in the ventricular cavities, and it is included in the cerebrospinal fluid existing in the subarachnoid space.

On pathological conditions, a supplementary sector occurs, and it is represented by the newly added volume (tumor, hematic collection, etc.), which develops in any sector, compressing and moving the fluids from their normal sectors.

The circulation of the intracranial fluids is secured by the cardiac activity that maintains the cerebral blood flux due to the pressure gradient:

$$MAP - ICP$$

where MAP is the mean arterial pressure and ICP represents the intracranial pressure.

The systolic arterial expansion induces a reshaping of the cerebral parenchyma and induces the motion of the cerebrospinal fluid from the ventricular system towards the spinal canal and towards the cranial subarachnoid space. According to the systolic-diastolic phases, there is a cyclic movement of the cerebrospinal fluid, and its circulation is not unidirectional, but pulsatory, with a reflux movement in the cardiac diastole.

The circulation of the intracranial fluids also involves the respiratory movements, which refers to the inspiration with thorax aspiration and the effect on the big cervical veins, as well as the movements of the ependymal cilia from the ventricular system.

The intracranial fluid circulation accomplishes several circuits:

- the bringing arterio-venous blood circuit: arteries – parenchymatous capillaries – veins
- the arterio-venous blood circuit that produces the cerebrospinal fluid: arteries – capillaries from the choroid plexuses – veins
- the metabolic exchange circuit of the interstitial fluid, at the level of the parenchymatous capillary: the arterial end of the capillary – parenchyma – the venous end of the capillary.
- the circuit of the cerebrospinal fluid, from the choroid plexuses to the resorption at the level of the venous sinuses.

These circuits are of the longitudinal circulation, entry – exit type.

- the trans-ependymal mutual circuit of the interstitial fluid – cerebrospinal fluid, which represents a communication with the other circuits.

This circuit accomplishes a transversal circulation, and it has a variable amplitude compared to the other circuits, in order to secure an optimal functioning of the intracranial hydrodynamics.

The circulation within every circuit is secured by the pressure gradient between the origin place and the resorption place of that particular fluid, and it depends on the flow resistance of the fluid.

References

[1] Arjmandi A, Liu K, Dorovini-Zis K. Dendritic cell adhesion to cerebral endothelium: role of endothelial cell adhesion molecules and their ligands.J Neuropathol Exp Neurol. 2009; 68(3):300-13.

[2] Damasio H. Human Brain Anatomy in Computerized Images, Edition: 2, Oxford University Press, 2005

[3] Depreitere B. Sectional Anatomy of the Human Brain, ACCO, 2000

[4] Fix JD Neuroanatomy , Edition: 4, Lippincott Williams and Wilkins, 2007

[5] Hamm S, Dehouck B, Kraus J, et al Astrocyte mediated modulation of blood-brain barrier permeability does not correlate with a loss of tight junction proteins from the cellular contacts. Cell Tissue Res. 2004 ;315(2):157-66.

[6] Iencean St M , Ciurea AV Intracranial hypertension : Classification and specific conditions of decompensation, Asian Journal of Neurosurgery, 2008, 3; 25-35

[7] Nakagawa S, Deli MA, Kawaguchi H et al.A new blood-brain barrier model using primary rat brain endothelial cells, pericytes and astrocytes. Neurochem Int. 2009 ;54(3-4):253-63.

[8] Netter F H Atlas of Human Anatomy, Edition: 4. Saunders Elsevier, 2006

[9] Melgar MA, Rafols J, Gloss D, Diaz FG. Postischemic reperfusion: ultrastructural blood-brain barrier and hemodynamic correlative changes in an awake model of transient forebrain ischemia. Neurosurgery. 2005 ;56(3):571-81.

[10] Mihailoff GA, Briar C. Nervous System, Elsevier Health Sciences, 2005

[11] Poller B, Gutmann H, Krähenbühl S et al The human brain endothelial cell line hCMEC/D3 as a human blood-brain barrier model for drug transport studies.J Neurochem. 2008,107(5):1358.

[12] Redzic ZB, Malatiali SA, Craik JD, Rakic ML, Isakovic AJ. Blood-brain barrier efflux transport of pyrimidine nucleosides and nucleobases in the rat. Neurochem Res.2009; 34(3):566

[13] Sandoval KE, Witt KA. Blood-brain barrier tight junction permeability and ischemic stroke.Neurobiol Dis. 2008 Nov;32(2):200-19

[14] Saunders NR, Møllgård K. Development of the blood-brain barrier.J Dev Physiol. 1984 ; 6(1):45- 57.

[15] Scarabino T, Salvolini U et all. Atlas of Morphology and Functional Anatomy of the Brain Springer, 2006

[16] Syková E, Nicholson C. Diffusion in brain extracellular space. Physiol Rev.2008 88(4):1277

[17] Thompson EJ. Proteins of the Cerebrospinal Fluid: Analysis and Interpretation in the Diagnosis and Treatment of Neurological Disease, Edition: 2, Academic Press, 2005

[18] Vemula S, Roder KE, Yang T, Bhat GJ et al. A functional role for sodium-dependent glucose transport across the blood-brain barrier during oxygen glucose deprivation.J Pharmacol Exp Ther. 2009 ;328(2):487-95.

[19] Zheng W, Chodobski A. The blood-cerebrospinal fluid barrier. CRC Press, 2005

Chapter III

Intracranial Pressure

1. General Considerations

The intracranial pressure is the intrinsic pressure developed by the endocranial-spinal structures (nervous parenchyma, blood and cerebrospinal fluid), as a result of the tensional (expanding) forces that the intradural content exercises on the limiting dural cover; its variations reflect the relationship between the cranio-spinal content changes and the capacity of accommodation to a supplementary volume.

The volume and distribution of water in the cranio-spinal space represent the most important factors for the intracranial pressure. The cranio-spinal space, which includes the skull continuing into the spinal canal, is a closed cavity with a viscous-elastic content represented by the nervous parenchyma, blood and the cerebrospinal fluid. The elastic properties of the nervous parenchyma, together with the blood vessels and the circulation of the cerebrospinal fluid allow an initial transitory accommodation to a supplementary volume, before the intracranial pressure increases. {5, 10,12,18]

The intracranial pressure values that are considered normal are between 2 mm and 12 mm Hg (with maximum normal values of up to 15 mm Hg), corresponding to values of 80-150 mm H_2O (the relationship is 136 mm H_2O = 10 mm Hg). (The pressure values are related to the atmospheric pressure, which is considered to be the zero value.) The normal ICP values are lower in infants, with maximum values of approximately 10 mm Hg. The normal intracranial pressure may also have negative values, depending on the position of the body or of the head, or it may register large increases for extremely short periods of time (during sneezing, etc.).

The intracranial pressure is considered to be high when it exceeds the value of 20 mm Hg, which is considered to be the normal limit ICP value.

The pressure measuring unit is the ratio of the unitary force acting to the unitary surface, therefore $1 \text{ N} / \text{m}^2$, and the IS pressure-measuring unit is Pascal (Pa):

$$1 \text{ Pa} = 1 \text{ N} / \text{m}^2,$$

and a kilopascal (kPa) is the equivalent of 7.5 mm Hg or of 102 mm H_2O.

The relationship between the cranium and the cerebral content has been postulated as constant by Monro (1783) and Kellie (1824): the intradural endocranial volume is constant and its content, made of the brain and, its blood content, is incompressible. At first, no one took account of the existence of the cerebrospinal fluid as an endocranial compartment, and, in 1846, Burrows introduces the idea of the mutual exchanges between the blood circulation and the cerebrospinal fluid. At the beginning of the past century, Weed and McKibben (1919, 1929) finalize the concept of the mutual exchanges among all the endocranial components. The Monro-Kellie outlook of the intracranial volume is considered valid for all the three endocranial components: brain, blood and the cerebrospinal fluid. Any variation of volume in one of the three components is immediately compensated by changes in the volume of the other components.

The cranial dural space is continued by the spinal dural sac; this allows small variations of capacity through the circulation of the cerebrospinal fluid. Moreover, the cerebral volume may vary due to changes of the blood vessels.

The endocranial content is made up of:

- the cerebral parenchyma: 80 % - 83.5 %, of which approximately 10% is made up of represented by the extracellular parenchymatous fluid,
- the cerebrospinal fluid: 10 %,
- blood and cerebral vessels: 7 % - 10 %.

and, as a principle, it is considered that:

Parenchymatous volume + Cerebral blood volume + Volume of the cerebrospinal fluid = Constant

According to the Monro-Kellie theory, any change in the volume of an endocranial component is followed by a compensatory reply from the other components in order to maintain the constancy of the endocranial volume. Each of the three normal intracranial components is incompressible. The fluid component of the cerebral parenchyma, which refers to the extracellular or interstitial fluid, the cerebrospinal fluid and the blood, moves physiologically, and, when the volume of an endocranial component increases, the fluid dynamics allows the volume change. Thus, an increase in the cerebral parenchyma volume should be followed by a decrease in cerebrospinal fluid volume or in the cerebral blood volume. However, the need to ensure a constant cerebral blood flux necessitates the increase in blood pressure in order to surpass the intracranial obstacle in case of an intracranial pressure increase. [10,12,16,17,18]

When a new extra-parenchymatous volume appears, its expansion occurs at the expense of the pre-existing normal volumes, and, if the expansion is slow, the volume variations is initially offset by the compression of the cerebral parenchyma.

The slow parenchymatous expansion continues to generate the decrease in the cerebrospinal fluid volume, the expansion being offset by an increased resorption or by the decrease in the secretion of the cerebrospinal fluid.

A rapid intra-cerebral or extra-cerebral expansion compresses and moves the cerebral parenchyma with ventricular collabation and the compression of the sanguine vessels, and it induces a rapid increase in the intracranial pressure once the compensating capacities have been exceeded.

In this case, the formula for the constant intracranial volume becomes:

Constant intracranial volume = Cerebral parenchymatous volume + Blood volume + Volume of cerebrospinal fluid + Supplementary pathological volume

This constant volume implies a fixed volume of the container, which is not valid in the case of a child with non-ossified sutures, where the modifications of the endocranial volume may induce an increase in the neurocranium volume. [10,18,21,22,23,24,30]

2. Intracranial Pressure Relationships

The fluid components (blood and cerebrospinal fluid) have pressure values that allow their circulation and the accomplishment of their physiological role; the blood pressure may vary around the average normal values of 100 mmHg, with accepted maximum values of up to 150 mmHg, while the pressure of the cerebrospinal fluid is of approximately 10 mmHg. In normal circumstances, these pressure relationships are maintained by complex and efficient mechanisms, especially in case of arterial pressure variations. [11,14,21]

The nervous parenchyma is considered incompressible and the intracranial pressure changes cause variations for the fluid components so that the ICP may be maintained within normal limits. The nervous parenchyma has a solid component, with a quasi-constant volume and a fluid component represented by the intracellular fluid and by the fluid from the interstitial space. The cellular content encloses water in metabolically active structures, and it has membrane delimitations, while the extracellular space contains the interstitial (interglial) fluid; normally, there is a hydrostatic and osmotic pressure equilibrium between these two compartments.

The composition of the interstitial fluid is the same as that of the cerebrospinal fluid and the parenchymatous pressure is in equilibrium with the pressure of the cerebrospinal fluid in the ventricular system and the sub-arachnoid spaces.

The parenchymatous pressure consists of the pressure of the cellular component (neurons and glia) and the pressure of the parenchymatous extracellular fluid. Normally, the pressure of the cellular component is constant and the variations in parenchymatous pressure are in caused by the pressure of the interstitial fluid.

The intracranial blood vessels (precapillary arterials) participate in the creation of the intracranial pressure in a pulsatory way via the great vessels and then by the permanent transmural pressure transfer towards the surrounding nervous parenchyma. The vascular pressure component is added to the intrinsic parenchymatous pressure value, so that the parenchymatous pressure is actually the result of summing the arterial pressure component with the pressure of the parenchymatous fluid:

Parenchymatous pressure = Vascularly induced pressure + Pressure of the parenchymatous fluid = Interstitial pressure

The resulting interstitial pressure is equal to the pressure of the ventricular or sub-arachnoid cerebrospinal fluid and identifying any of these values gives the value of the intracranial pressure. [12,21,23,29]

ICP = Parenchymatous interstitial pressure = Pressure of the cerebrospinal fluid

Starting from the previously given formula of the cerebrospinal fluid resorption (see CSF Resorption):

$$\text{CSF resorption rate} = \frac{\text{Pressure gradient (CSF – Venous sinus)}}{\text{Flow resistance}}$$

and considering the fact that, in normal circumstances, the secretion of the cerebrospinal fluid is equal to its resorption, it follows that:

$$\text{CSF production} = \frac{\text{Pressure gradient (CSF – Venous sinus)}}{\text{Flow resistance}}$$

which leads to the intracranial pressure = the pressure of the cerebrospinal fluid:

CSF pressure = CSF production x Flow resistance + Venous pressure in the sagittal sinus

or **ICP = CSF production x Flow resistance + Venous pressure in the sagittal sinus**

The vascular participation in ICP is limited by the mechanical behaviour of the arterial wall and it is underlined by the tension component of intracranial pressure waves.

The ICP value is diurnally variable depending on position, type of activity, circadian variations of the cerebrospinal fluid production, various physiological situations etc.; there are also individual variations.

The classification of the increased ICP must be made by assessing the intracranial pressure – duration fluctuation, which is schematically characterized by a relation of inverse proportionality. The intracranial pressure variations are considered normal, depending on the duration of the various ICP values.[12,29,30]

The cerebral sanguine circulation is ensured by the difference between the sanguine pressure and the intracranial pressure. The cerebral perfusion pressure, designated CPP, is calculated according to the formula:

CPP = MAP – ICP

where MAP represents the average blood pressure.

The mean arterial pressure (MAP) is an average blood pressure and it is defined as the average arterial pressure during a single cardiac cycle. At normal resting heart rates MAP can be approximated using the more easily measured systolic and diastolic pressures, SP and DP:

$$MAP \simeq DP + \frac{1}{3}(SP - DP)$$

or equivalently

$$MAP \simeq \frac{(2 \times DP) + SP}{3}$$

and it has an approximate value of 95-100 mmHg.

MAP is the perfusion pressure seen by organs in the body and it is considered that a MAP greater than 60 mmHg is enough to sustain the organs .

As an individual gets older or as the vascular elasticity diminishes, the MAP increases progressively, getting closer to the value of the systolic arterial pressure.

Starting from the MAP value, the cerebral blood flow, CBF, may be assessed, as it is related to the cerebral perfusion pressure and the resistance of the cerebral vessels to the sanguine flow:

CBF is equal to the cerebral perfusion pressure (CPP) divided by the cerebrovascular resistance (CVR):

CBF = CPP / CVR

or

CBF = (MAP – ICP) / CVR ,

where CVR represents the cerebral vascular resistance.

The supply of a uniform cerebral sanguine flow is fundamental for cerebral functioning.

In normal circumstances, the intracranial pressure is smaller, less than 8 - 10 mm Hg, and the mean arterial pressure (MAP) may oscillate, sometimes significantly.

The complex auto-regulating mechanisms of the cerebral circulation ensure a cerebral perfusion pressure of minimum 70 mm Hg and the cerebral blood flow is maintained normal at quasi-constant values of 50 – 65 ml / 100 g / min.

The intracranial pressure is the result of summing the blood pressure component and the parenchymatous fluid pressure, and it is manifested as a pulsatile pressure. On the intracranial basic pressure background , the ICP recording reveals the waves that corresponds to the pulsations of the cerebral vessels, the respiration or the pressure variations induced by the physiological activities (miction, coughing etc.).

The volume-intracranial pressure relationship depends on the limited endocranial and spinal volume and on pressure variations.

The dural cranio-spinal space is divided into four sectors with different volumes, by means of the dural prolongations and by the cranial and spinal anatomic shape:

- the supra-tentorial space, the one with the largest volume, and which is partially segmented by the brain scythe in the two supra-tentorial compartments, each of them corresponding to a cerebral hemisphere,
- a cranial sub-tentorial compartment (posterior cerebral fosse);
- a spinal compartment that communicates with the intracranial space via the occipital hole.

The pressure relationships in this communicating system with a fixed volume are established by the pressure transmission between neighbouring compartments in order to equalize pressure.

The volume-pressure physiological changes of one of the intracranial compartments (brain, blood content, cerebrospinal fluid) cause a compensatory reply from the others in order to maintain a constant ICP value.

The relationship between the intracranial volume (sum of the component volumes) and ICP is underlined by the concept of the compliance of the intracranial content.

Cerebral compliance is the ability of the brain to adapt to changes in volume (dV) inside the cranium in order to reduce changes in pressure (dP) and it is defined as the volume variation per pressure unit (the volume variation generated by the pressure variation of 1 mm Hg).

$$C = dV / dP$$

The inverse relationship is defined by the cerebral elastance, E:

$$E = dP / dV$$

A brain is compliant if a large change in ventricular volume results in a small change in ICP.

In 1978 Marmarou introduced the pressure volume index (PVI) : the theoretical volume, which is required to increase the measured ICP up to 10-fold ; normal value 25-30 cc.

The PVI is evaluated with either a defined volume load dV (eg. injection of fluids in positioned ventricular catheter, inflating of an epidural balloon) or withdrawal (eg. CSF drainage via ventricular catheter) and simultaneous measuring of the baseline pressure (Po) and maximum pressure (Pp):

$$PVI = \frac{V}{\lg \frac{P_p}{P_o}}$$

The experiments run by Langfitt on monkeys and the subsequent human studies have established that the intracranial volume-intracranial pressure relation has a specific phase behaviour, which is revealed on the pressure recordings :

- during the first stage, the small and constant increases in the intracranial volume do not cause pressure changes;
- the intracranial volume changes that continue to occur at the same growing rate, determine a progressively accentuated pressure increase,
- at a given moment, the continuing intracranial volume increase with the same variation causes a sudden rise of the pressure curve with an exponential aspect.

During the first two stages of the intracranial volume-intracranial pressure variation, there is a significant cerebral compliance: there may be a relatively high increase in the intracranial volume and a small increase in the intracranial pressure. There is a point when the compliance equals the elastance, which means that the unitary volume variation corresponds to a unitary pressure variation, after which the cerebral compliance decreases and any intracranial volume variation corresponds to a significant pressure increase.

The intracranial pressure value for which the cerebral compliance is equal to the cerebral elastance, is a value that has features of a maximum limit, a value up to which the volume-pressure regulating mechanisms still have compensatory capacities.

Monitoring of the intracranial pressure has allowed the identification of normal values, of the limit values that correspond to the compensating possibilities, as well as of pathological ICP values; the normal and abnormal aspects of the ICP charts have also been established.

The normal intracranial pressure has values of less than 10 mm Hg; negative ICP values do not have a pathological significance because, when ICP is measured, the zero value corresponds to the atmospheric pressure. The high ICP values may occur for a short period of time in certain physiological circumstances (coughing, sneezing, defecation, etc.) with no implications on the cerebral parenchyma. When ICP increases beyond 20 mm Hg, it is considered to be pathologic, and it requires a treatment based on the duration of the high pressure values.

In order to keep the morpho-functional integrity of the cerebral parenchyma, it is necessary for the cerebral perfusion pressure to be maintained at appropriate values relative to the intracranial pressure.

The pressure equilibrium is unstable, and the comparison between the MAP and ICP values reveals the CPP variations; the permanent auto-regulating mechanisms of the cerebral circulation rapidly intervene and maintain the CPP at normal values, it being the most important parameter of the nervous functioning.

3.Intracranial Pressure Waves

The intracranial pressure recording shows the intracranial pressure waves, as a manifestation of the arterial and venous pulsations that are intracranially transmitted with the quasi-constant background of intracranial pressure under normal circumstances. The intracranial pressure wave has an ascendant path, corresponding to the arterial pulsation; this is the anacrotic wave, or the percussion wave, P_1; it is continued by the returning wave, which reflects the cerebral compliance, noted by P_2 , with a descending path under normal circumstances, i.e. normal ICP values and a compliant cranium; a small incisure follows, corresponding to the dicrotic wave or the venous pulsation, noted by P_3. On the intracranial pressure background, which corresponds to the P_2 value, the vascular tension oscillations are added, as they lead to the pressure increase - P_1, and then to its decrease - P_3. [6,11,13,28]

The normal aspect of ICP waves ispresented in figure 17.

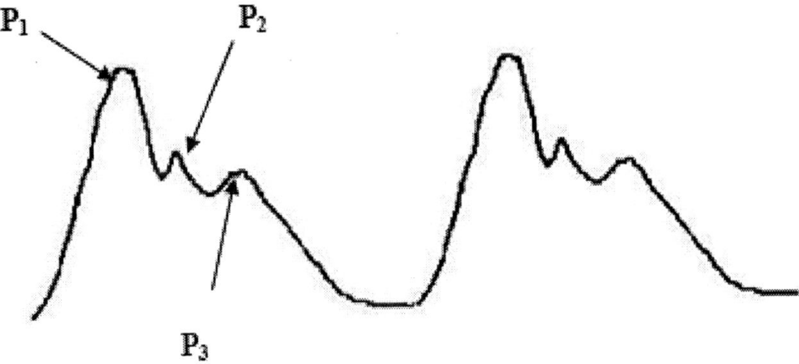

Figure 17. Normal intracranial pressure waves:

P_1 - is the anacrotic wave or the percussion wave, corresponding to the arterial pulsation,
P_2 - corresponds to the ICP value, in case of normal compliance,
P_3 - the dicrotic wave, which corresponds to the venous pulsation

This is how the intracranial waves appear in a normal cerebral compliance situation. In the case of increased ICP values, the cerebral compliance is reduced, and the aspect of the intracranial pressure waves is modified:

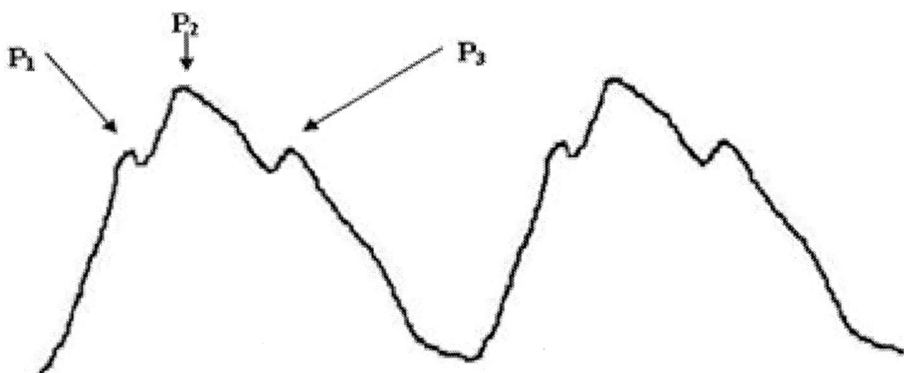

Figure 18. Increased intracranial pressure waves,

It is obvious that P_2 has a higher value than P_1, which corresponds to a cranial cavity with a decreased compliance or to a non-compliant one.

The ICP monitoring shows the intracranial pressure increases, with changes in the aspect of the ICP waves that correspond to the decrease in cerebral compliance:

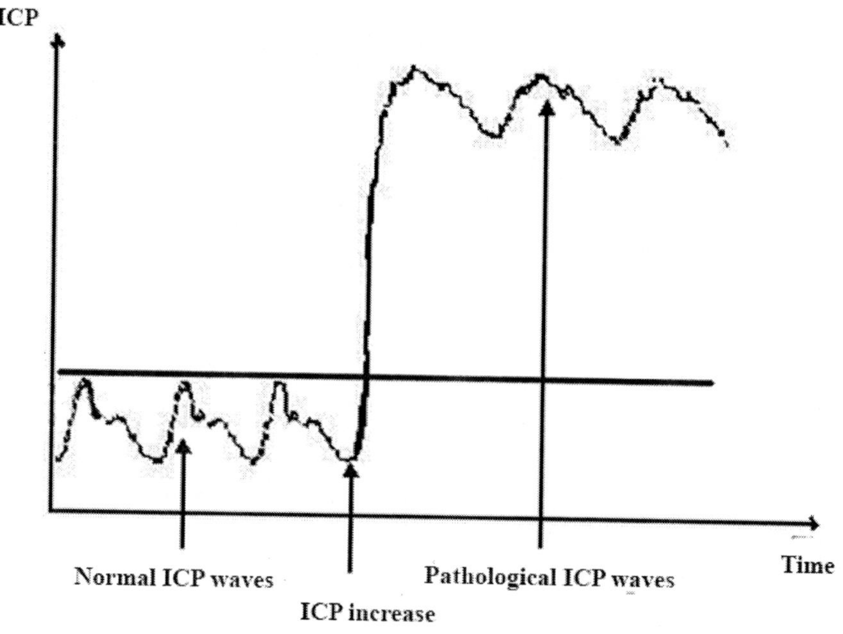

Figure 19. ICP recording revealing the pressure increase and the modified forms of the waves .

Lundberg presents the graphical aspects noticed during the pathological recording of intracranial pressure:

- plateau waves or pressure waves of type A, which correspond to certain cyclic increases in ICP with the aspect of a plateau, up to values of 50 mm Hg (sometimes 50 – 100 mm Hg), and a duration of 5 to 20 minutes. The ICP increase, due to various causes, produces the decrease in the cerebral perfusion pressure, and, therefore, the reaction consists of an auto-regulating mechanism via cerebral vasodilatation; in the case of a very low or absent cerebral compliance, ICP continues to increase. Therefore, A waves occur as a reaction to the cerebro-vascular autoregulation because of the decrease in the cerebral compliance, and their presence announces a decompensation with clinical aggravation.
- B waves, which represent ICP variations with variable amplitude, of 20 mm Hg on average, (20 – 50 mm Hg) or more, for several minutes (usually 1 – 2 minutes); they may occur in groups, or they may announce the occurrence of the A waves. B waves are thought to be caused by the fluctuation of the cerebral blood flux, which induces changes in the intracranial blood volume. They correspond to a decrease in the cerebral compliance, reaching the limit of the compensating capacities of an ICP increase. However, it has been statistically established that, in the case of a traumatic

coma, the presence of B waves may be followed by a clinically favorable development.

- C waves, which are related to the arterial pressure variations, they do not exceed 20 mm Hg, and they are considered normal.

The parameters of these waves are sometimes difficult to define, and there is a tendency to use a descriptive presentation: plateau waves, waves with the frequency of 1/ min, etc.

Lundberg's findings are considered classical, but it is currently believed that the intracranial pressure values are normal or increased depending on the period when the ICP increase occurs and on the duration of these values. They are significant for the cerebral functioning based on the capacity of maintaining the cerebral perfusion pressure.[11,28]

Clinical data have established that every patient presents individual variations of ICP values and of the cerebral perfusion pressure values, but intracranial pressure values of more than 20 mm Hg are thought to be pathological, and their rapid decrease is required.

4. Intracranial Pressure Increase

The intracranial pressure increase may occur in physiological circumstances for very short periods of time due to the increase in the venous blood volume in one of the following cases: coughing or sneezing effort, expiration effort with the closed glottis (defecation effort, labor expulsion effort), in positions of the body with the head downwards, etc.. The intracranial pressure increase may also occur in other circumstances unrelated to a cranial-cerebral pathology, such as high intensity pain with different locations. [3,12,14,24]

In pathological circumstances, if the compensating mechanisms for ICP increase reach their limit, a small increase in the intracranial volume causes an exceeded compensating possibility, leading to intracranial hypertension. This alteration of the ICP controlling mechanisms may occur in certain predisposing conditions, which allow the anticipation and prevention of the intracranial hypertension decompensation.

Such situations include:

- expansive intracranial processes: tumors, hematomas (subdural, extradural, intra-parenchymatous), intracranial abscesses
- diffuse brain edema due to: disorders in the auto-regulation of the cerebral circulation in traumatic brain injury, encephalitis, asphyxia, or due to the cytotoxic brain edema in traumatic brain injury, intoxications, etc.
- blocked CSF circulation in hydrocephalus, expansive intracranial processes, meningitis

The following values are accepted for the normal and pathological intracranial pressure:

- the normal intracranial pressure has values of up to 10 mm Hg; there may be negative ICP values without a pathological meaning;
- the intracranial pressure with values of 10-15 mm Hg is also thought to be within normal limits. In the case of a cerebral traumatic pathology, these values require

close monitoring as the intracranial pressure equilibrium is unstable, and various situations – coughing, change in the patient's position, aspiration of the tracheal-bronchial secretions, visitors' presence, etc., may bring about ICP increases to values of up to 5 - 8 mm Hg, which leads to a final intracranial pressure with values of more than 20 mm Hg.

- In the case of values between 15 - 20 mm Hg, the cerebral function is not significantly affected. These ICP values represent a pressure range that corresponds to the compensating limits and to a high degree of instability in pathological situations. Pressure changes are caused by small variations of intracranial volume (brain edema, supplementary intracranial volume) and they can still be compensated by changes in the cerebrospinal fluid and the blood circulation.
- above 20 mm Hg, ICP is thought to cause cerebral lesions, depending on how long these increased values last. The compensating mechanisms are no longer possible, and the ICP values increase rapidly, leading to movements of the cerebral parenchyma (pressure cones), while the decrease in the cerebral perfusion pressure causes the occurrence of irreversible ischemic lesions. [11,14,27]

The intracranial pressure is thought to be increased when the pressure values are maintained within the 15 - 20 mm Hg range, with the limit of 20 mm Hg, or when pressure waves are present in the plateau (A waves) or grouped B pressure waves.

Depending on the increasing speed of intracranial pressure and on the type of lesion that has caused the pressure change, the effect is either the cerebral substance movement, i.e. the occurrence of pressure cones with the direct compression of the parenchyma and the local circulatory disorder, or the decrease in the cerebra perfusion pressure due to exceeded auto-regulating mechanisms of the cerebral circulation with generalized cerebral suffering and cerebral ischemia.

Acute and supra-acute lesions, caused usually by severe cerebral traumatisms,cause a large ICP increase with decompensation due the occurrence of brain herniation. Progressive intracranial hypertension syndromes, including traumatic ones, bring about disorders of the cerebral circulation and the decrease in the cerebral perfusion pressure.

Characteristics of Intracranial Pressure Increase

The intracranial pressure increase is specific for every pathogenic mechanism of cerebral illnesses, and the ICP monitoring reveals characteristic features that establish the clinical evolution of the intracranial hypertension [11,13,24, 29]:

- the speed of the increase in intracranial pressure up to the normal limit values of 20 mm Hg and above this value: therefore, there are two segments of the ICP increase:
    1. pressure increase segment up to the normal limit
    2. pathological pressure increase segment, up to the maximum value
- the maximum pathological value reached by the intracranial pressure,
- duration of the pathological intracranial pressure maintenance,

- the period of recovery to normal pressure values
- the frequency of pressure increase reoccurrence or the frequency of remissions.

Several types of pressure increases may be described based on the above-mentioned characteristics and on the clinical evolution:

1) the supra-acute intracranial pressure increase with rapid decompensation. The intracranial pressure increase is very rapid up to the value of 20 mm Hg, and afterwards to a maximum pressure value. This pressure increase occurs in supra-acute cases of intracranial hematoma, of traumatic brain edema, or in the extending edema of the malignant middle cerebral artery syndrome, when a supplementary volume develops rapidly at the intracranial level. The infraclinical period is very short and the intracranial hypertension decompensation is accelerated due to the high speed of the increase in the supplementary intracranial volume and to the exceeding of the compensating capacities. The Pressure increases very rapidly and the pathological values of the intracranial pressure are of up to 30 - 40 mm Hg. These pathological values are maintained for a short while due to the rapid decompensation.

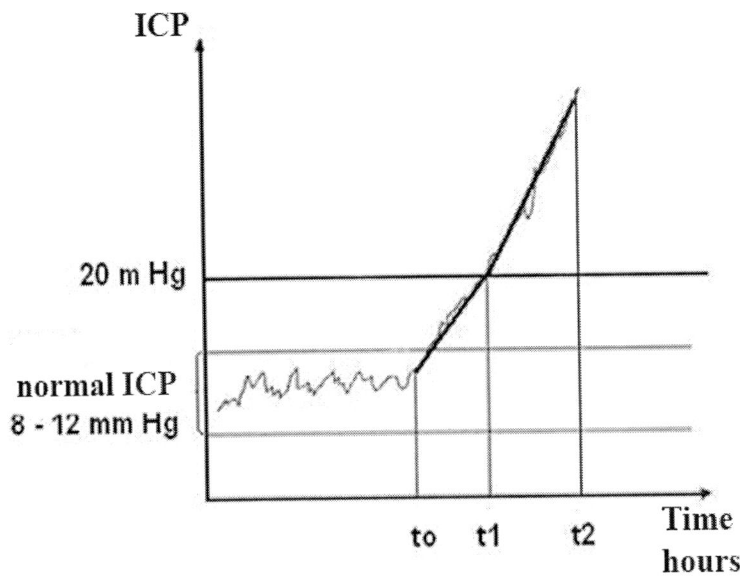

Figure 20. Supra-acute intracranial pressure increase; intervals to-t1 and t2-t1 are short, of a few hours .

2) acute intracranial pressure increase, preceded by a long infraclinical period. In these cases, the intracranial pressure reaches and exceeds the normal pressure values over a long period, with a slow speed of intracranial pressure increase. This is the type of intracranial pressure increase that occurs in cerebral tumors, cerebral abscesses, chronic subdural hematomas, etc., usually when the occurrence and development of

the supplementary intracranial volume progresses slowly. During the infraclinical period, the compensation of the pressure increases caused by the newly added volume occurs, reaching the limit value. Once the compensating capacities have been exceeded, the intracranial pressure increase is rapid up to the maximum values, which are of approximately 30 - 40 mm Hg. The duration of these pathologic pressure values is short due to the rapid decompensation.

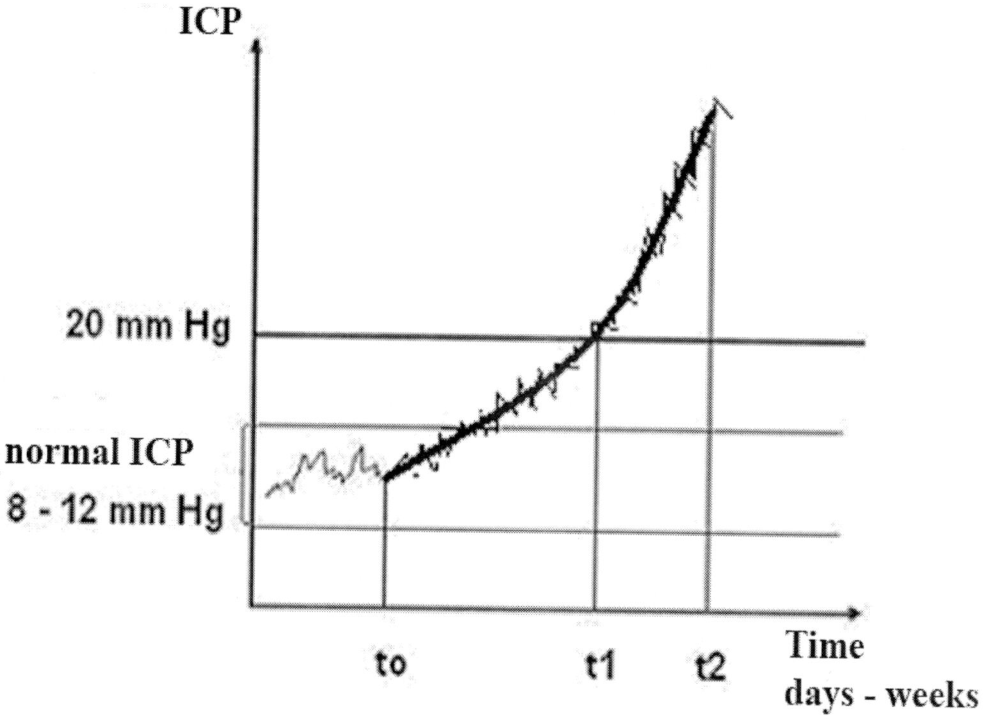

Figure 21. Acute ICP increase, with a prolonged infraclinical period and a rapid decompensation; the interval to-t1 is prolonged, it may last for weeks or even months, and the decompensation lasts for a few days.

3) the acute increase, with a short infraclinical period and a longer period of pathological pressure increase. The intracranial pressure increase to the normal limit of 20 mm Hg is rapid but slower than the supra-acute pressure increase. Once the normal pressure values have been exceeded, the ICP increase is gradual, but at a slower speed compared to the previous period. It reaches pathological pressure values of approximately 30 mm Hg. This occurs in hypertensive encephalopathy, which includes a self-limiting mechanism: the intracranial pressure increase caused by the blood pressure increase and the occurrence of the cerebral vasodilatation eventually lead to the collabation of the intracranial sanguine vessel walls, with the decrease to a certain degree in the cerebral sanguine volume. It is clinically manifested as an incomplete or complete intracranial hypertension syndrome, which

may be decompensated unless appropriately treated. The period when the pathological ICP values are maintained depends on the efficiency of the etio-pathogenic therapy of the high blood pressureand on the pathogenic therapy of the ICH syndrome.

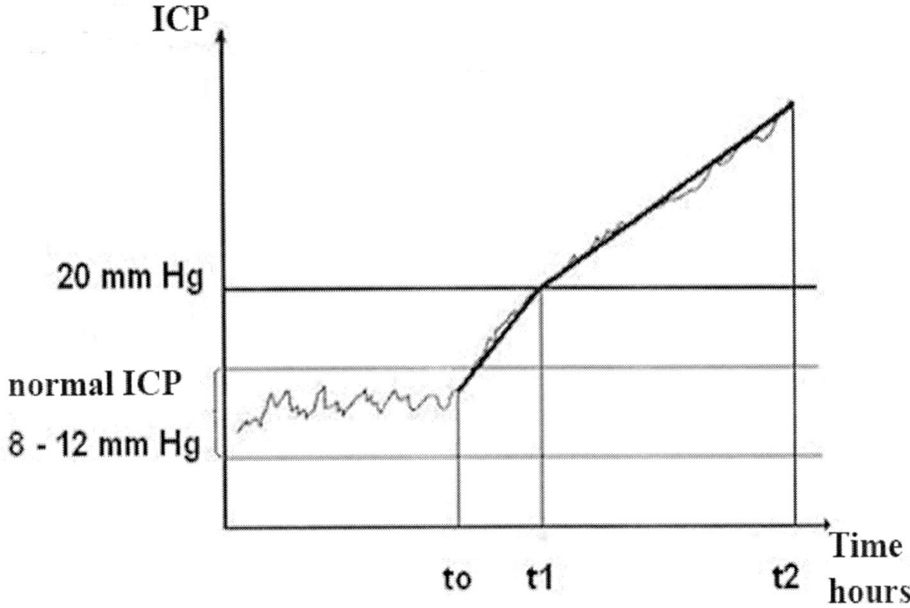

Figure 22. Acute ICP increase, with a short infraclinical period, and a prolonged period of the decompensation risk; the interval to-t1 is short, of a few hours; the interval t1-t2 is prolonged.

4) slow intracranial pressure increase with a prolonged infraclinical period and a long period of pathological ICP increase. This type of pressure increase occurs in cases of diminished resorption of the cerebrospinal fluid in acute meningitis, sub-arachnoid hemorrhage, cerebral venous thrombosis and thrombosis of dural sinuses, cerebral thrombophlebites etc. Intracranial pressure increases slowly and gradually until it reaches the normal limit value of 20 mm Hg, and it continues its slow increase with periods when it returns to normal pressure values, according to the etiology of the ICH syndrome. The compensating capacity of the pressure increase allows a prolonged maintenance of the cerebral sanguine flux, and the duration of the pathological pressure values is rather long. There is a development towards a prolonged, complete or incomplete ICH syndrome, without leading to clinical decompensation.

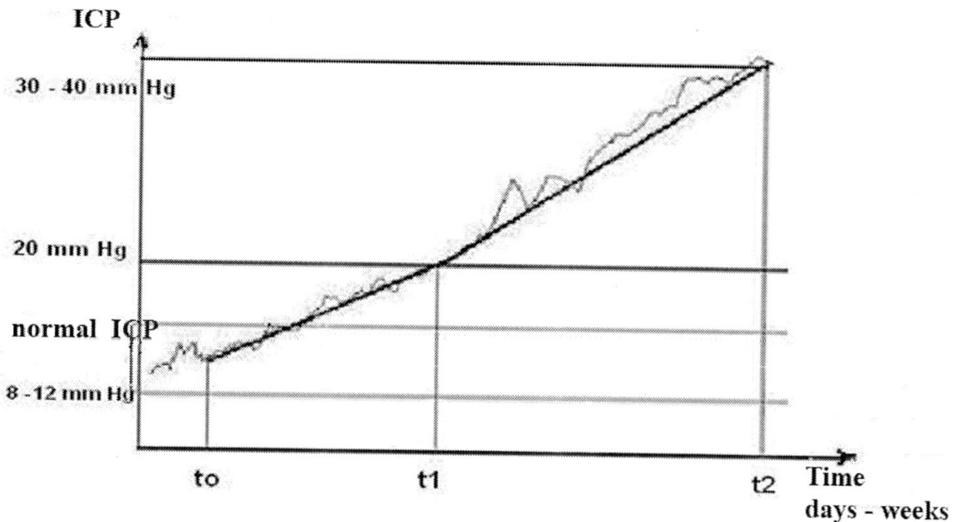

Figure 23. Slow ICP increase, with a long infraclinical period and a prolonged period of pathological pressure values.

5) the "chronic", extremely slow increase in intracranial pressure. This occurs in cases of idiopathic intracranial hypertension and in certain cases of thrombosis of intracranial venous sinuses. A very slow intracranial pressure increase occurs, which allows good pressure compensation and the maintenance of the cerebral sanguine flux at almost normal values. The pathogeny of the idiopathic intracranial hypertension syndrome is complex, but the intracranial pressure increase has a "chronic" aspect. The pathogenic ICP values are very high, reaching to 60 - 80 mm Hg; these are valuesd that may be maintained in a plateau for long periods of time. There is a clinical evolution towards an incomplete ICH clinical syndrome, with no decompensation.

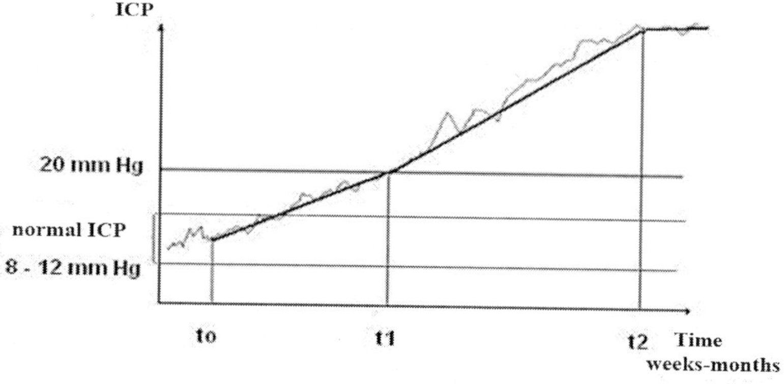

Figure 24. Chronic ICP increase, with prolonged infraclinical period and an extremely long period of pathologic pressure values.

5. Compensating Mechanisms

The occurrence of intracranial volume modifications leads to the initiation of compensating mechanisms in order to prevent intracranial pressure increase. Compensating mechanisms act during the period when there is a significant cerebral compliance, which means that supra-unitary values are reached. Supra-unitary cerebral compliance shows that the intracranial space is not completely occupied by the solid parenchymatous volume, and that there are possibilities of dislocating the intracranial fluid components, that is the sanguine content, the cerebrospinal fluid and the extracellular parenchymatous fluid, which may allow the expansion of the supplementary component. [12,16,17]

The compensating possibilities are physically limited by the volume of the intracranial space that is occupied by the fluid components, and they are physiologically limited by the need of minimal sanguine volumes and circulating CSF volumes that ensure the cerebral functioning.

The acting period of the compensating mechanisms corresponds to the variation interval of intracranial pressure between the values of 15 - 20 mm Hg, and the compensating mechanisms have maximum efficiency when ICP reaches the approximate value of 20 mm Hg.

Pressure compensation has few mechanisms available:

- pressure equalization in all compartments;
- progressive and discrete ICP increase up to values that to not hinder the normal cerebral functioning; from a normal average of less than 10 - 12 mm Hg, ICP increases to 15 - 20 mm Hg;
- depending on the intracranial component of interest (nervous parenchyma, blood content, CSF), a pressure decrease attempt may occur in the other sectors due to the decrease in the volume of that particular sector

The pressure compensation is limited by the short interval that is accessible to compensation and by the rapid variation from the normal ICP to the pathological ICP.

The volume compensation may be more efficient, depending on the applied mechanism, and it also depends on the speed of the occurrence and development of the supplementary intracranial volume, but it is limited by the fixed cranial volume.

The volume-compensating mechanisms are as below:

- collapsed nervous parenchyma due to the compression of the neighbouring structures by the supplementary volume,
- distension of dura mater by using the extradural cranio-spinal elastic reserve space (the buffer space), that is: intracranially, at the level of the cavernous sinuses and at the level of the spinal dura mater, which is surrounded by fat and voluminous venous plexuses, which can be rapidly emptied (in a minute).
- fluid spaces are emptied due to the compression and obliteration of the basal cisterns and to a faster cranio-spinal fluid circuit,

- significant decrease in the blood content (between 3 % and 10 %) in several minutes, maintaining though the cerebral perfusion pressure.

These mechanisms are prompt, but they have a limited effect due to the fixed volume in which the volume extension may occur.

- increase in the CSF resorption: due to the very large fluid absorption reserve, a drainage of up to 100 – 200 ml per hour may occur in the case of intracranial pressure increase, (the average CSF secretion is of 20 ml / hour in circadian rhythm)
- decrease in the hydric content of the directly compressed cerebral parenchyma, due to the increase in the resorption of the interstitial fluid, especially in the case of expansive processes with slow compression.

These two mechanisms are progressive and slow, but their efficiency is much higher.

The considerable increase in the resorption of the cerebrospinal fluid is one of the means used to accomplish the complex maintaining mechanism of fluid fluxes (blood and fluid fluxes) in the case of idiopathic intracranial hypertension. [12,17,29]

The compensating process of the intracranial pressure increase includes all the mechanisms, and it has a unitary development. From the moment when the volume-pressure disorders occur, leading to the cerebral compliance decrease, all these mechanisms become active: they are initiated rapidly and concomitantly, and their effect is summed-up. This provides a compensating period, and, from a therapeutic point of view, may allow the identification of the cause, as well as its solution.

The continuation of the supplementary volume expansion causes the intracranial pressure increase, the above-mentioned reply mechanisms continue their activity, but they no longer ensure the ICP decrease, and nervous parenchyma movements occur due to the pressure gradient among the cranial-spinal compartments: collapsed ventricles, unilateral hemispheric edema, median ax movement, and the other brain herniations. The brain herniation is a pressure equalizing mechanism among the cranio-spinal compartments; it involves the slide, traction and compression of nervous structures with severe neurological disorders. The traction, as well as the slide or shearing of planes initially occur at the level of the moved nervous structure, then the local brain edema is continued by the compression of a limiting rigid anatomic formation or / and the mutual compression with the local nervous structure where the movement has taken place. Local ischemia occurs afterwards, as well as the softening of the nervous formations involved.

The rapid development of the supplementary intracranial volume causes a sudden increase in the intracranial pressure, while the compensatory mechanisms prove to be inefficient with decompensation by means of pressure cones. The progressive development of the supplementary intracranial volume allows a longer compensation period, with a gradual exhaustion of all the compensatory mechanisms and a final decompensation, unless a therapeutic intervention has occurred.

6. Intracranial Pressure Measurement

Intracranial pressure is the pressure developed in the endocranio-spinal structures (nervous parenchyma, blood and CSF), and is caused by the expansion forces of the content on the limiting dural covering layer.

After the lumbar puncture was introduced by Quincke at the end of the 19th century, the pressure of the lumbar CSF is measured by lumbar puncture. In a horizontal position, the pressure of the ventricular CSF is equal to the pressure of the lumbar spinal CSF, and, obviously, when sitting, the intra-ventricular pressure is lower than the pressure of the lumbar CSF. In adults, the normal pressure of the lumbar CSF is of approximately 100 – 200 mm H_2O. [1,2,7,25]

The arguments that have excluded the lumbar manometry are the risk of brain herniation in the case of certain expansive intracranial processes, which could not be discovered before the existence of the modern explorations, and the possibility that the spinal CSF pressure may not always accurately reflect the intracranial pressure (in the case of the blocked CSF circulation). The measurement of the intracranial pressure by means of lumbar puncture is currently accepted as an exploration and a diagnosis criterion in idiopathic intracranial hypertension (after the exclusion of an endocranial lesion by CT or a cerebral MRI).

Nowadays, the ICP measurement is done via invasive means, which establish a connection through a trepan hole between the endocranial space and the exterior measuring system (transducer – pressure sensor), which also records the ICP values. There are also various attempts at ICP monitoring using non-invasive procedures, which do not involve the used of the trepan hole.

In the case of the invasive methods, the pressure transducer (or the pressure sensor) may be extra-cranial and it has a fluid connection to the endocranial fluid space, or the pressure sensor is introduced at the endocranial level. [1,4,7,8,9,25,26]

The pressure measuring systems that share a fluid coupling may be the following ones:

- intra-ventricular catheter,
- sub-arachnoid screw (or bolt),
- subdural catheter,
- epidural catheter.

The measuring systems with intracranial pressure sensor are:

- intra-ventricular pressure sensor,
- intra-parenchymatous pressure sensor,
- subdural pressure sensor,
- epidural pressure sensor.

The pressure sensor may be placed practically anywhere in the intracranial space, but the ICP values may be different precisely due to the sensor's location being different to the intra-ventricular position. Moreover, the ICP values may have a different sector development, depending on the location of the pathological process that replaces the intracranial space.

The external pressure sensor shares a fluidic coupling with an intracranially placed catheter – in the lateral ventricle, at a subarachnoid or extradural level. The external pressure sensor may be recalibrated (brought to the zero pressure value), and it must be fixed at the same level as the patient's head, in order to avoid any possible errors. The obstruction of the intracranial catheter or of the fluidic connection with the extracranial pressure sensor may also lead to ICP measuring errors.

The intracranial pressure measuring systems must comply with several conditions:

- the pressure measuring limits must range between 0 – 100 mmHg;
- the accuracy of the measurement and the maximum accepted error: the accepted error must be of less than 1 mm Hg within the value interval 0 – 20 mm Hg and, in the interval 20 – 100 mm Hg, the maximum accepted error must not exceed 5 %. According to other authors, the precision of the measurement must be of ± 0.1 mm Hg for the interval 0 – 10 mm Hg, and of ± 1.5 mm Hg up to 100 mm Hg. [1,18,25,26]

Intra-Ventricular Catheter

The ICP establishment and monitoring by means of the intra-ventricular catheter is the most precise and safe method, and it represents the reference value of intracranial pressure. The intra-ventricular catheter has a fluidic connection to the extracranial pressure sensor, and it allows both the ICP measurement and the CSF external drainage. The pressure sensor may be easily calibrated and recalibrated; this calibration secures the accuracy of the ICP calculation.

Usually, the catheterization of the lateral ventricle is performed on the part of the non-dominating cerebral hemisphere; there are studies that have revealed sector pressure increases based on the location of the intracranial lesion, recommending the ICP measurement in the cerebral hemisphere that is controlateral to the lesion, especially for the lesions of the temporal lobe.

The advantages of this method are:

- the most accurate measurement of the intracranial pressure value,
- the possibility of CSF external drainage with therapeutic purpose, as an immediate ICP decreasing measure, and for laboratory measurements. Moreover, the ventricular catheter allows the intra-ventricular introduction of medication when needed.
- the possibility of an easy recalibration of the pressure sensor, without changing the ventricular catheter.
- the cost of the sensors is more advantageous.

The disadvantages of this method refer to:

- the risk of infection, which ranges from 3.6 % to 7 %. It has been noticed that the infectious risk may vary in the case of the ICP monitoring during the first days, but it does not continue to increase in the case of a monitoring that lasts for more than 5 days.

- the intra-ventricular catheter or the fluidic connection to the external sensor may be obtruded (blood or cerebral detritus).
- the lateral ventricles may be collapsed in the case of significant brain edema, and the introduction of the ventricular catheter may be difficult.

The Subarachnoid Tubular Screw (Subarachnoid Bolt)

The subarachnoid screw or bolt is a cylindrical metallic device with an external thread that is fixed by means of a trepan hole on the side of the non-dominating cerebral hemisphere at the level of the subarachnoid space. The device has a fluidic connection by means of a column of sterile physiologic serum with the external pressure sensor. The Richmond (or Becker) screw is the most used one, but there are other variants too (the Ledds screw, the Philly screw).

It is easily installed, the infectious risk is much more reduced than in the case of the ventricular catheterization, and, moreover, there is no need for the ventricular location for the catheter. The subarachnoid screw may be obstructed by blood or by the brain edema; moreover, the ICP values that are thus established are less accurate than the other methods.

It is a procedure that is extremely easy to set up and monitor.

Subdural Catheter

The subdural catheter is introduced in the subdural space by means of a trepan hole, and it forms a fluidic coupling by means of a physiologic serum column (or the Ringer solution) with the external pressure sensor. This procedure does not allow the CSF drainage, and erroneous values may occur due to the compressive effect of dura mater on the catheter; moreover, the collected pressure waves are of a poor quality. The procedure is less and less used.

The Fiber Optic Intracranial Pressure Sensor

Pressure sensor catheters have been developed starting from the intra-vascular transducers: the pressure is measured by a sensor placed on the top of a fine catheter, prolonged by an optic fiber that transmits the intracranial pressure values. The external diameter of the catheter is of only 1.3 mm.

The catheter is calibrated before the insertion and it can not be recalibrated afterwards, unless it is associated to a ventricular catheter.

The system does not depend on a fluidic coupling with the exterior, and the recording does not depend on the position of the external sensor relative to the patient's head.

The fiber optic intracranial pressure sensor can be introduced in the ventricle, in the subdural space, by means of the Richmond tubular screw or directly at the intra-parenchymatous level. As it does not allow the CSF drainage, most frequently it has an intra-parenchymatous insertion, and it is often called the intra-parenchymatous sensor.

The pressure values determined using the intra-parenchymatous sensor are close to the ones determined by means of a ventricular catheter, the differences ranging from 1 to 4 mm Hg.

The advantages of the intra-parenchymatous sensor system with optic fiber reside in the easy insertion, a reduced rate of infections, the independence of the values read regardless of the head position, and the ability to continue the monitoring as the patient is transported.

The disadvantages of this procedure are the impossibility of CSF drainage, as an emergency therapeutic operation in ICP increase, and the impossibility of performing laboratory explorations; this sensor catheter can not be recalibrated, which means that the catheter must be changed in case of a disorder; moreover, the optic fiber is rather fragile. These systems are gradually becoming more and more used.

Non-invasive procedures for intracranial pressure measurement

Various non-invasive procedures of intracranial pressure measurement have been proposed, some of them being quite clever, but they have not been used in current practice as they are rather complicated, they are too expensive, or they have not been completely validated yet.[1,8,15,22]

The first non-invasive ICP measurements have been calculated in new-born infants and young children based on the epicranial measurement of the pressure transmitted at the level of the anterior fontanel; the procedure is not applicable after the closure of the fontanel.

The best known procedures that have been experimented and compared to the ICP reference data are:

- the ICP assessment based on the acoustic or dielectric cranial-cerebral properties: reflection of acoustic waves on the cranial bone – endocranial space interface; measurement of the cranial dielectric modifications at high-frequency currents (1-1.5 MHz), etc.
- intracranial pressure measurement by establishing the movement and the tension of the tympanum,
- venous ophthalmo-dynamometry,
- ICP measurement near the jugular bulb using an intravascular catheter that is introduced in the jugular vein with a small balloon and a pressure sensor,
- the tissue resonance analyzing method: it consists of the analysis of the relationship between the frequencies produced by the reflection of an ultrasound signal against the wall of the 3rd ventricle and the cardiac cycle.
- the ICP measurement using the method of the MRI is quite difficult to apply in clinical practice.

Choice of Monitoring System

Although the ICP monitoring using the intra-ventricular catheter represents an accurate measurement, which allows the establishment of an intracranial pressure reference value, the fiber optic intracranial pressure sensor is increasingly used due to its easy installation. The main disadvantages are the fact that it can only be calibrated at installation.

The monitoring system is chosen based on the characteristics of each particular case:

- intra-ventricular monitoring is preferred in situations when a ventricular drainage might be needed,
- in cases of a significant brain edema, with collapsed cerebral ventricles, a subdural catheter or a fiber optic intracranial pressure sensor is used.
- in cases of post-surgery monitoring, if dura mater is closed, a subdural catheter may be used, or, better yet, an intra-parenchymatous sensor catheter.

The best ICP monitoring procedure is based on the intra-ventricular catheter that can allow the CSF drainage when needed, and the monitoring system can be recalibrated. The catheter obstruction incidents can be easily solved, and the infectious risks can be controlled.

References

[1] Adelson PD, Bratton SL, Carney NA, Chesnut RM,et al Intracranial pressure monitoring technology. Pediatr Crit Care Med. 2003 ;4(3 Suppl):S28-30.

[2] Asil T, Uzunca I, Utku U, Berberoglu U. Monitoring of increased intracranial pressure resulting from cerebral edema with transcranial Doppler sonography in patients with middle cerebral artery infarction. J Ultrasound Med. 2003 ;22(10):1049-53.

[3] Bershad EM, Humphreis WE 3rd, Suarez JI. Intracranial hypertension.Semin Neurol.2008 ;28 (5):690-702.

[4] Chesnut RM. Intracranial pressure monitoring in brain-injured patients is associated with worsening of survival. J Trauma. 2008 ;65(2):500-1

[5] Czosnyka M, Czosnyka ZH, Richards HK, Pickard JD. Hydrodynamic properties of extraventricular drainage systems. Neurosurgery. 2003 Mar;52(3):619-23.

[6] Czosnyka ZH, Cieslicki K, Czosnyka M, Pickard JD. Hydrocephalus shunts and waves of intracranial pressure. Med Biol Eng Comput. 2005 Jan;43(1):71-7.

[7] Forsyth R, Baxter P, Elliott T. Routine intracranial pressure monitoring in acute coma.Cochrane Database Syst Rev. 2001;(3):CD002043.

[8] Frischholz M, Sarmento L, Wenzel M, Aquilina K, Edwards R, Coakham HB. Telemetric implantable pressure sensor for short- and long-term monitoring of intracranial pressure.Conf Proc IEEE Eng Med Biol Soc. 2007; 514.

[9] Geeraerts T, Newcombe VF, Coles JP et al. Use of T2-weighted magnetic resonance imaging of the optic nerve sheath to detect raised intracranial pressure. Crit Care. 2008;12(5):R114.

[10] Iencean St M A new classification and a synergetical pattern in intracranial hypertension Medical Hypotheses , 2002 ;58(2):159-63.

[11] Iencean St M Pattern of increased intracranial pressure and classification of intracranial hypertension. Journal of Medical Sciences, 2004, 4, 1 :52- 58

[12] Iencean St M , Ciurea AV Intracranial hypertension : Classification and specific conditions of decompensation, Asian Journal of Neurosurgery, 2008, 3; 25-35

[13] Jetzki S, Kiefer M, Eymann R, Walter M, Leonhardt S. Analysis of pulse waves in intracranial pressure. Conf Proc IEEE Eng Med Biol Soc. 2007 ;2863-6.

[14] Kalmar AF, De Ley G, Van Den Broecke C et al. Influence of an increased intracranial pressure on cerebral and systemic haemodynamics during endoscopic neurosurgery: an animal model British Journal of Anaesthesia 2009 102(3):361-368

[15] Kimberly HH, Noble VE. Using MRI of the optic nerve sheath to detect elevated intracranial pressure. Crit Care. 2008;12(5):181.

[16] Kurtcuoglu V, Poulikakos D, Ventikos Y. Computational modeling of the mechanical behavior of the cerebrospinal fluid system. J Biomech Eng. 2005 ;127(2):264-9.

[17] Levine DN. Intracranial pressure and ventricular expansion in hydrocephalus: have we been asking the wrong question? J Neurol Sci. 2008 15;269(1-2):1-11.

[18] Marmarou A, Bullock R, Avezaat C et al (eds) Intracranial Pressure and Neuromonitoring in Brain Injury: Proceedings of the Tenth International ICP Symposium, Williamsburg, May 25-29, 1997, Springer Wien New York, Birkhäuser, 1998

[19] Marshall LF. Pediatric traumatic brain injury and elevated intracranial pressure. J Neurosurg Pediatr. 2008 ;2(4):237-8

[20] Mayer SA, Coplin WM, Raps EC. Cerebral edema, intracranial pressure, and herniation syndromes. J Stroke Cerebrovasc Dis. 1999 ;8(3):183-191.

[21] Miller MM, Chang T, Keating R, Crouch E, Sable C. Blood flow velocities are reduced in the optic nerve of children with elevated intracranial pressure. J Child Neurol.2009; 24(1):30-5.

[22] Minns RA . Problems of Intracranial Pressure in Childhood, Cambridge University Press, 1991

[23] Penn RD, Lee MC, Linninger AA, Miesel K, Lu SN, Stylos L. Pressure gradients in the brain in an experimental model of hydrocephalus.J Neurosurg. 2005 ;102(6):1069-75.

[24] Piper I, Barnes A, Smith D, Dunn L. The Camino intracranial pressure sensor: is it optimal technology? An internal audit with a review of current intracranial pressure monitoring technologies.Neurosurgery. 2001 ;49(5):1158-64.

[25] Poca MA, Martínez-Ricarte F, Sahuquillo J et al . Intracranial pressure monitoring with the Neurodur-P epidural sensor: a prospective study in patients with adult hydrocephalus or idiopathic intracranial hypertension. J Neurosurg. 2008 ;108(5):934-42.

[26] Sedý J.The rapidity of intracranial pressure increase reflects the grade of neurogenic pulmonary edema. J Clin Anesth. 2008 ;20(6):479

[27] Stevens SA, Stimpson J, Lakin WD, et al. A model for idiopathic intracranial hypertension and associated pathological ICP wave-forms. IEEE Trans Biomed Eng. 2008 ;55 (2 Pt 1):388-98.

[28] Wakeland W, Goldstein B. A review of physiological simulation models of intracranial pressure dynamics. Comput Biol Med. 2008 ;38(9):1024-41.

[29] Walters FJM Intracranial Pressure and Cerebral Blood Flow, Physiology, 1998,8,4:1-4

Chapter IV

Pathogenesis of Intracranial Hypertension

1.General Data

The occurrence and evolution of intracranial hypertension are determined by the pathological volume changes in the three intracranial components (cerebral parenchyma, cerebrospinal fluid and blood circulation), depending on the etiology and the individual compensation capacities of the intracranial pressure increase. [2,11]

The primary pathogenic mechanisms of the intracranial hypertension are:

- the increase in the volume of a normal intracranial component without the corresponding decrease in the volume of the other two components
- the occurrence of a supplementary endocranial volume.

The main endocranial component is the cerebral parenchyma, and its volume increase refers to an intrinsic parenchymatous increase that has a compressive effect on the other two intracranial components. The occurrence of a supplementary intracranial extra-parenchymatous volume has a compressive effect on all the other three intracranial components. [11,13,21]

The extrinsic compression of the parenchyma may be caused by:

- an extra-parenchymatous space-replacing process:
  - sub-dural, extra-dural hematoma, etc.;
  - extra-cerebral tumor: meningioma, neurinoma, etc.,

or there is

- a compression of the parenchyma by means of
  - a ventricular compressive expansion in the internal obstructive hydrocephalus of various etiologies.

The variations of the intrinsic parenchymatous volume may occur by means of several mechanisms:

- the change in the volume of certain normal structures – significant vasodilatation (brain swelling)
- parenchymatous volume change due to a cerebral, diffuse or localized edema
- the occurrence of certain space-replacing intra-parenchymatous lesions: intra-cerebral hematoma, tumors, abscesses, etc.
- mixed traumatic lesions: brain lacerations.

The brain edema is a parenchymatous response during the development of any of the above-mentioned mechanisms. Moreover, the changes in the endocranial components vary for every type of mechanism. [11,14,25,42]

From a schematic perspective, the pathogeny of the intracranial hypertension may be presented as follows:

I. Modification of the normal endocranial components:

A. brain parenchyma:

- brain edema, of any type and by any mechanism,
- hyper-secretion of cerebral interstitial fluid in idiopathic ICH

B. cerebrospinal fluid:

- hyper-production (in idiopathic ICH through the transfer of the excessive parenchymatous interstitial fluid towards the cerebrospinal fluid or, rarely, in tumors of choroid plexus)
- resorption decrease

C. cerebral vascularization:

a.- arterial component:

- the systemic high blood pressure with hydrostatic brain edema (the cerebral blood flow remains constant due to the increase in the cerebral perfusion pressure)
- the increase in the cerebral blood flow through the decreased vascular resistance in hypercapnia, etc.

b. – the venous component: low venous draining with:

- decrease in the resorption of the cerebrospinal fluid
- venous stasis

II. The creation of a compressive (supplementary) volume:

D. extrinsic compression (outside the parenchyma)

- extra-parenchymatous intracranial expansive lesion (sub-dural, extra-dural hematoma, meningioma, neurinoma, etc.)
- parenchyma compression due to the expansion of the ventricular system (congenital hydrocephalus, by ventricular tumor, tumor of the posterior fosse).

E. supplementary parenchymatous intrinsic volume:
- expansive process – tumor, intra-cerebral hematoma, brain abscess

2. Modifications of the cerebral parenchyma

The cerebral parenchyma reacts to the occurrence and evolution of a supplementary intracranial volume via the following types of changes:

A. bio-mechanical

- local, neighbouring / sector compression,
- cerebral parenchyma movements,
- the added volume occupies the intracranial space and the compensatory capacity is exceeded

B. bio-chemical

- at the level of the vascular wall or
- at the level of the neurons and neuroglia,with the formation of the brain edema.

These disorders occur based on the characteristics of the intracranial space-replacing process (the nature and rapidity of the intracranial expansion, location, etc.) and they happen successively or concomitantly. [2,3,6]

Biomechanical Effects

The formation of a supplementary intracranial mass initially induces various mechanical effects on the adjacent tissues. Sometimes the parenchymatous metabolic changes are concomitant.

If the supplementary volume is extra-cerebral, it causes a local compression from the outside on the brain parenchyma, and, if the new volume develops in the cerebral substance, this neo-formation causes the compression of the surrounding tissues.

The extra-cerebral expansion continues at the same time as the brain substance movement and the reduction of the fluid spaces, causing the decrease in the volume compensating capacity. The parenchymatous compression is accentuated by the reduction of the extra-cellular space and by the decrease in the volume of the cells and nervous fibers, which corresponds to the disappearance of the volume-compensatory possibilities.

The directly compressed cerebral tissue experiences various cellular hypoxia phenomena, which cause metabolic modifications that induce the occurrence of the brain edema.

At this stage, the compensating mechanisms are exceeded, causing the ICP increase, which marks the beginning of the intracranial hypertension.

In the case of a new volume that develops in the cerebral substance, at first there is a neighbouring compression of the cerebral parenchyma (white, grey substance, vessels), and rapidly or concomitantly, there are disorders at the level of the adjacent vessels, as well as disorders in the metabolisms of the cells from the neighbouring cerebral sectors, with the development of the brain edema.

As the volume of the neo-formation grows and is accompanied by the increase in the perilesional edema, the cerebral substance is pushed and moved, filling all the free spaces and exhausting the compensating capacity, the ICP begins to grow and the intracranial hypertension starts. [3,6,21,23,27]

The resulting conclusion is that, in the case of an extra-cerebral intracranial expanding process, the parenchymatous biomechanical effects occur at first until the volume-compensating mechanisms are exceeded, then the brain edema occurs with the ICH development; in the case of an intra-cerebral neo-formation, the local compressive effect is simultaneous to the occurrence of the brain edema, and then, with the contribution of the edematous compression, the biomechanical effects are completed, the compensating possibilities are exhausted, and the intracranial hypertension is installed.

The ICH evolution is influenced by the pathogenic characteristics of the newly-added volume:

- the nature of the supplementary volume (hematoma, benign, malignant tumor, etc.), which determines the evolution of the lesion, i.e. the speed of the volume increase and the conditions of the perilesional edema
- the degree of cerebral distortion (the compression and the movement of the cerebral structures with cerebral herniation)
- the location of the new volume with the possibility of blocking the circulation of the cerebrospinal fluid (the location at the level of the hemispheric poles is accompanied by a delayed ICH syndrome, etc.)

As far as the pathogenic stages are concerned, the newly added volume exhausts the volume compensation at first, and then it generates the ICP increase. Therefore, ICH is brought about by the increase in the intracranial volume, with a manifestation of the disequilibrium on the capacity of the skull, which translate into a pressure conflict.

The most serious consequences of the ICP increase are the effect on the cerebral perfusion pressure, which causes the cerebral ischemia, and the sector pressure differences between the cranial-spinal compartments, with the possibility of a cerebral hernia.

Brain Edema

The brain edema represents a non-specific cerebral reaction to a very large number of factors that induce disorders of the brain-blood barrier, and determine the increase in the hydro-electrolytic content of the cerebral parenchyma with water accumulation and an increase in its volume. [3,21,29,30]

The brain edema may occur due to changes in intracranial volume, as an immediate or delayed reaction in the evolution towards ICH, or the brain edema may be secondary to another cause (inflammatory, metabolic, allergic, hypoxia, etc.), causing the increase in the cerebral parenchyma volume with biomechanical and pressure changes that are characteristic to the evolution of the intracranial hypertension syndrome.

The brain edema is:

- an intermediate stage in the evolution of the intracranial pressure disorders towards ICH
- it represents a first stage in the conflict volume – intracranial pressure, identifying the ICP increase.

This etiopathological relationship, with the participation of the brain edema at various moments in the evolution towards ICH, is involved in the differentiation of the four types of intracranial hypertension (parenchymatous, vascular, meningeal and idiopathic).

The importance of the brain edema in cerebral reactivity is so significant because it represents a common pathogenic element or it occurs as a complication in many neurosurgical, neurological or medical conditions.

Brain Edema Pathogenesis and Types of Edema

The brain edema is the response of the cerebral parenchyma to various aggressions, while the mechanisms that produce the abnormal intracellular and interstitial hydro-electrolytic – protein accumulation are complex and they represent alterations of the normal membrane transporting mechanisms (capillary and glio-neuronal). [21,27,30,32]

At the level of the central nervous system, the volume of the extra-cellular space is of approximately 10 - 12 % (sometimes it may exceed 15 %) and it is limited by the glial cells (practically, it consists of the inter-glial spaces, the inter-glio-neuronal and inter-glio-endothelial fissures).

Astrocytes (astroglia) present numerous end-feet that cover the surface of the neuronal entities (somatic neurilemma), forming the perineural sheath, and surrounding the terminal arterioles and the capillaries. At this level, the glial prolongations have the classical aspect of astrocytes end-feet and, by apposition, they form the pericapillary sheath. The lateral adhesion between the glial vascular prolongations forming the pericapillary sheath sometimes also allows direct exchanges between the capillary endothelium – interglial space.

At the level of the white substance fibers, there are oligodendrocytes (oligodendroglia), which form the myelin sheath and the pericapillary sheath for the white matter-vessels.

The neuron is not in contact with the capillary because the glial cells and the extracellular matrix are interposed between the two structures, mediating all the exchanges and taking part in forming the brain-blood barrier.

The capillary endothelium is made up of the cells that limit the capillary lumen, tightly connected by impermeable junctions (occlusion junctions) that hinder the passage of the ions and molecules from the capillary lumen.

The movement of substances from the capillary lumen at the level of the pericapillary sheath happens only by means of a membrane transport, so that the vascular endothelium represents a barrier with selective permeability. The perithelial cells (pericytes) surround the vascular endothelium from place to place, as they are enclosed in the basement membrane. The endothelial contact with the glial end-feet happens by means of the basement membrane, and the interposed pericytes represent an intermittent doubling of the brain-blood barrier.

The transport circuit is continued by the circulation through the extracellular matrix and on the intra-glial way to and from the neuron, where the glio-neuronal communication through the peri-neuronal sheath is achieved. [33]

The membrane permeability and the transport depend on the membrane and cytoplasm pH, on the oncotic pressure in the above-mentioned compartments, on the membrane electric charge, on the cytoplasm and extracellular enzymes, the ionic calcium concentration, etc., factors that regulate and secure the transport selectivity.

The capillaro-glial, glio-interstitial and glio-neuronal exchanges include all transport methods: diffusion for gas and small molecules, facilitated diffusion , active transport ,osmosis, transport of macro-molecules by transcytosis etc.

The transport mechanisms have a different kinetics, some of them having a sufficiently high developing speed (for example, the molecule of Na^+- K^+-ATP-ase may be divided in up to 100 ATP molecules in one second) ensuring the continuity of metabolic processes.

Water transport depends on the concentration gradient and/or on the difference of hydrostatic pressure between neighbouring compartments.

The intracellular osmotic pressure and the cellular volume are regulated by ionic transport systems, and water circulation is achieved by membrane water channels. The water motion balances the osmotic pressure between the capillary lumen – endothelium – astrocyte – glial interstice – neuron, participating in the maintenance of the pressure equilibrium in the cerebral parenchyma. [6,21,34]

These micro-transport means ensure a normal neuronal functioning and metabolism through the permanent transport of substances and the energetic transfers.

The membrane and intracellular capillary-glial-neuronal exchanges depend on numerous factors and they may be slightly disturbed, but the multitude of transfer types allows the partial compensation of disequilibrium, if this disequilibrium is a limited one.

The alteration of the cellular transport mechanisms depends on the type of aggression: specific or not, local or extended, and, at first, it may mainly affect only one transfer system with subsequent extension, or it may be generalized from the beginning.

The cellular response (endothelial, glial and neuronal) depends on the type of aggression and on the compensating capacity by activating or blocking the non-affected transport systems. Exceeding the cellular compensation abilities induces a blockage of the communication between the affected cells and the normal ones at the level of the extracellular matrix, causing a local delimitation and isolation.

This mechanism is not very efficient due to the histological and functional characteristics of the cerebral parenchyma: the astrocyte has numerous prolongations that participate in the formation of the pericapillary sheaths for several capillaries or of the same capillary in several areas, and, similarly, the perineural prolongations correspond to several neurons.

Exceeding this compensation by isolation is caused by an aggression of high intensity or with a prolonged action, which extends the disorder of the cerebral parenchyma. [3,6,33,40]

The neuronal functioning (generation and transmission of the action potential) imposes the existence of a circuit of contribution and metabolic elimination:

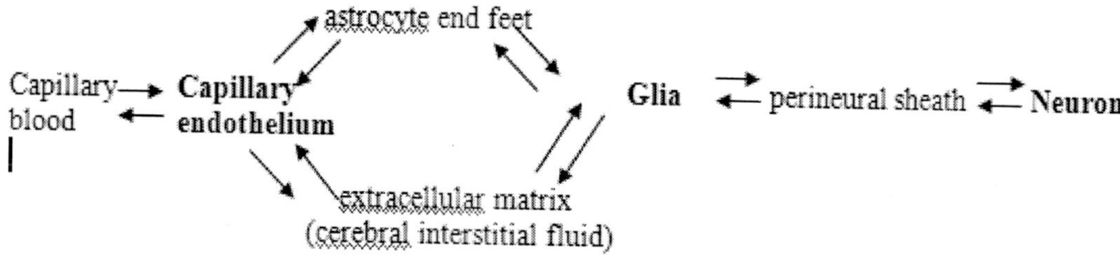

Figure 25. Scheme of the metabolic neuronal circuit, underlining the central role of neuroglia.

The disorder or the interruption of these metabolic circuits constitutes the start of the pathogenic mechanism of the brain edema because it represents the first stage of water accumulation at an intracellular and/or extracellular level. A further disorder occurs generated as the local compensating possibilities are exceeded. During the extension stage, the cellular/extracellular participation is specific and it is determined by the lesional characteristics.

The edema continues to propagate, and it covers larger territories of cerebral parenchyma.

The installation and development of the brain edema follow several stages:

- initiation of the disorder related to the glial-neural metabolic circuit by an alteration of the transport mechanisms;
- local extension, when the characteristic cellular / extracellular lesion is defined;
- progression based on the interest manifested by progressively larger areas of parenchyma.

From a classical perspective, several mechanisms that generate the brain edema have been differentiated, depending on the type of the aggression that causes the edema initiation and the cellular lesional characteristics from the local extension phase. [21,33,41,42]

Usually, there is not one type of brain edema, but several that mingle because, during the edematous extension phase, there is a conversion of the compartments that are not involved at the beginning by an indirect effect.

The hydro-electrolytic and/or protein accumulation can happen at the intracellular level and/or in the extracellular matrix (interglial space), which differentiates three types of brain edema:

- cellular (glio-neuronal)
- extracellular

- mixed, when the intersection between the two compartments is almost equal, simultaneous from the beginning, or the edema may involve only one area at the start and it includes both of them afterwards.

Usually, the brain edema begins either at an intra- or at an extra-cellular level, and, during its evolution, it is propagated to the other sector; therefore, the initiation and the extension correspond to a particular type of edema, and, during the progression phase, the edema becomes a mixed type one based on the ample intersection of the parenchyma.

The differentiation in types of cellular, extracellular or mixed brain edema is determined by specific initiation factors, it happens through individual pathogenic mechanisms, and it has a predominant location in the territories of the cerebral parenchyma where the support for the pathologic action prevails: increased cellularity in the grey matter where mostly the cyto-toxic cellular edema appears, and a more reduced cellularity, with ampler intercellular spaces in the white matter, where especially the extracellular edema develops.

Cellular Brain Edema

Cellular brain edema or cytotoxic brain edema (Klatzo, 1967) , is the growth in the volume of the parenchymatous cellular elements: glial cells firstly, neurons and even endothelial cells later. It is an osmotic cellular edema. The beginning is brought about by different factors which alter the membrane exchanges and cause an increase in the osmotic pressure and then an increased intracellular liquid buildup. The membrane permeability for passive diffusion is altered and the enzymatic capacity for active ionic transport and transport of hydrosoluble molecules is reduced, thus causing an intracellular buildup of ions, water etc.. It occurs when the blood-brain barrier is intact. [2,3,4]

The cellular swelling and the disappearance of the interglial area occur first ; then the evolution continues through the decrease in the volume of the CSF and through vascular collapse.

This imbalance in the intra/extra cellular osmotic pressure is caused by:

- intracellular hyperosmotic pressure: - in hypoxia, anoxia, by blocking the physiological transport mechanisms; - osmotic imbalance syndromes (sometimes in diabetic ketoacidosis, hemo-dialysis) - neurotoxins [5,6],
- extracellular hypotonicity - acute plasmatic hypoosmotic pressure (water intoxication also known as hyper-hydration, inadequate ADH secretion).
- in intracerebral hemorrhage, thrombin produces brain injury via direct brain cell toxicity with intracellular hypertonicity and brain edema occurs.
- the dialysis disequilibrium syndrome : it is characterized by brain edema and neurologic deterioration. Two theories have been proposed to explain why this occurs: a reverse osmotic shift induced by urea ; and a fall in cerebral intracellular pH. The molecular basis for the dialysis disequilibrium syndrome is the connection of a reduced expression of urea transporter (UT-B1) and an increased expression of aquaporin (AQP4 and AQP9) in astrocytes. The urea exit from astrocytes during the rapid removal of the extracellular urea through hemodialysis ; as a result, urea transiently acts as an effective osmole, promoting intracellular water movement into the brain. ("brain intracellular acidosis" theory).[4,8,9,30]

- peudohypoxic brain swelling is characterized by a cellular brain edema and death of neurons after intracranial hypotension with decreased parenchymatous interstitial fluid and decreased cerebro-spinal fluid. MRI show hypodensities or altered intensities in the basal ganglia and/or thalamus. [17,20,37]

Cellular brain edema extension occurs in two stages:

(1) in the beginning, the glial edema with a narrowing of the extracellular space occurs; a compensation by temporarily increasing resistance to the water inflow is attempted , but the mechanism is overpowered .
(2) the glial cellular edema advances; it is followed by the neuronal edema and cellular decay caused as the glial membrane breaks , the edema fluid is exteriorized and the extracellular space increases. The cellular edema progresses through the transition from this local stage of extension and cellular injury beginning to the stage of affecting first the neighbouring parenchymatous areas and then further ones. Cellular brain edema develops generally at the gray matter level, but also in white matter, depending on cell density.[42,43,47]

Extra-Cellular Brain Edema

Extra-cellular brain edema (interglial or interstitial) appears as a result of the buildup of edema fluid – water, ions and proteins – in the extracellular space of the brain parenchyma. The extracellular space (extracellular matrix) is formed mainly of the space between the gliacytes. Its volume is considered to be 12-15% of the total brain parenchyma volume; it is composed of structural elements of the fundamental matter secreted by the glial cells and it has the metabolic roles of membrane stabilization and intercellular circulation of molecules with various functions (cellular growth factors, chemical mediators etc). Its part in the pressure balance is relatively low in normal circumstances and mainly limited to interglial colloid – osmotic pressure changes. The increase in the volume of the intercellular space occurs to the detriment of the glial cells and is caused by the buildup of fluid originating from the glial cells or from the structures that are covered by the glial cells (capillary vessels, ventricular cavity). Both the composition of the extracellular edema fluid and the extension method, in its evolution rapidity and its amplitude, vary according to the fluid's blood or ventricular origin. Depending on the origin of the edema fluid several mechanisms that generate extra cellular edema are described. [7,17,49] When the edema fluid has a blood origin the interglial buildup occurs by the modification of the transport mechanisms at the blood-brain barrier level: capillary endothelium crossing the pericapillary astrocytic foot processes or passing through the pericapillary glial extensions. When the edema fluid originates in the brain ventricles, it is represented by CSF which crosses the ventricle wall.

There are three types of extra-cellular brain edema :

A) Hydrostatic extra-cellular brain edema
B) Oncotical extra-cellular brain edema
C) Hydrocephalic extra-cellular brain edema

A. Hydrostatic Extra-Cellular Brain Edema

This type of brain edema (mechanism of ultrafiltration) can be caused by pronounced increases of intravascular brain pressure in severe high blood pressure.A difference in the hydrostatic pressure relative to the endothelial cells and then to the glial-extraglial pressure occurs. The ultrafiltration mechanism consists of the transcellulary passage of water, ions and substances with low molecular weight (glucose, small aminoacids) from the blood plasma due to the difference in hydrostatic pressure. The extension of this hydrostatic extracellular brain edema depends on the arterial pressure values and on the length of the high blood pressure accesses. The self regulatory mechanisms of brain circulation can function up to systolic arterial pressure values of 150 mm Hg. It is thought that this edema occurs when the brain blood barrier is intact.The hydrostatic brain edema covers the brain parenchyma diffusely, but it frequently affects the gray matter with a higher intensity. [27,29,33,46]

B.Oncotical Extra-Cellular Brain Edema

Oncotical extracellular brain edema (vasogenic edema) is caused by a endothelial capillary modification, generally known as an increase in the capillary permeability or open blood-brain barrier, and consists of the crossing of the endothelium by plasmatic molecules, water and ions, which accumulate in the extracellular space.

The macromolecules' transport mechanism is a fast transcytosis and this transport method at the brain capillary endothelium is pathological. This edema corresponds to a classic vasogenic edema and is a severe alteration in the blood-brain barrier. [8,9,10,11] Thus, it is thought that it occurs in the case of a so-called "open" blood-brain barrier. The beginning of endothelial transcytosis for plasmatic molecules can be caused by many factors, the first of which are the cytokines, which appear in many pathological states: brain tumours, inflammations, haemorrhages, brain infarcts. In malign brain tumours, the reactive glial cells generate endothelial kynases that cause endothelial proliferation with increased endothelial permeability. The proteins that cross the capillary endothelium cannot penetrate the astrocytes and pass through the glial extensions' connections, accumulating interglially. The extension of this edema type is brought about by the increase in extra cellular oncotic pressure simultaneously with a greater water and ions flow from the blood capillary. A complex ionic, hypoxic and energetic imbalance of the endothelial-cellular exchanges occurs, affecting the glioneuronal metabolism.

These injuries of a localized nature relative to the disorder that causes them grow step by step by expanding to the neighboring areas until the edema covers a large area. At this stage the brain edema has combined features, due to the existence of extracellular edema and the secondary beginning of cellular edema. Oncotically caused extracellular brain edema, known to be caused by a vasogen mechanism, is localized mainly in the cerebral white matter where the cells are fewer and intercellular spaces are larger and more extensible. [12,17,44]

C.Hydrocephalic Extra-Cellular Brain Edema

The extracellular edema (interglial) fluid originates from the brain ventricles and is composed of CSF which crosses the ventricle wall as a result of the increase in intra ventricular fluid pressure. It is an extracellular edema produced by the increased hydrostatic pressure mechanism from the brain ventricles.[12]

The low increase in the pressure of intra ventricular CSF leads to the acceleration of membrane exchanges with the periependymal glial cells .

In obstructive hydrocephalus ventricular CSF increases progressively with an increase in intra ventricular hydrostatic pressure and cavity expansion. The ependymal layer is tensioned, the ependymal cells stand out and CSF crosses the ependymal wall, shunting the limited membrane transport mechanisms. It is thought that periventricularly accumulated CSF is present predominantly in the extracellular space; it passes interglial, is transported and reaches the blood capillary simultaneously, creating a supplementary circuit for fluid removal which causes a general hypotony of the periventricular white matter. The beginning of the hydrocephalic edema is caused by increasing the hydrostatic pressure of CSF through obstructive hydrocephalus; the extension is made by widening the interglial space at the time of CSF's glial passage, and the development of the hydrocephalic edema occurs as a result of the ventricular distension.

The extracellular brain edema occurs as a result of an imbalance in extra cellular colloid – osmotic pressure through the following mechanisms:

1. the hypertony of the extracellular matrix increases and the endothelial permeability increases too :
    a. endothelial transcytosis = "vasogen" edema is the oncotically caused extracellular edema, and
    b. endothelial ultra filtration – hydrostatic extracellular edema, and
2. the hypotony of the glial cells increases: it is a hydrocephalic edema.

Mixed Brain Edema.

The mixed brain edema includes in variable ratios both types of brain edema, cellular and extracellular (mixed cytotoxic/vasogenic edema*)*; they can be present together from the beginning or can appear successively. When the two edema types evolve successively, the damage of one compartment reaches a limit and will bring about the other type of injury and they will evolve together and develop different features from either the cellular and the extra cellular edema. Usually there is no pure brain edema – only cellular or only extracellular, because between glial cells and the extracellular matrix there is an ionic and metabolic balance which represents a functional dependence. Neuronal edema depends on the glial changes and it is also influenced by the modifications in the extracellular matrix. In the case of vascular mechanisms that cause interstitial edema, glial metabolic and secondary neuronal derangements also occur.

The brain edema is combined almost from the beginning, one of its forms prevailing; this predominance could be just initial or it could be a prolonged predominance, depending on the edema's evolution. The concomitance of the glial and neuronal lesions and the simultaneous existence of the two edema types were ascertained and it is emphasized that in both situations the astroglia is a common element in the damage, hence in the combined brain edema the glial damage is considerable. [3,32,41,48]

The mixed brain edema occurs as a result of the causes that produce each brain edema type, either:

a. concomitantly – the two types coexist and evolve together from the beginning, or
b. successively – initially either of the cellular brain edema or the extra cellular brain edema occurs; during its evolution it leads to the appearance of the other type and it finally turns into the combined brain edema .

The typical mixed brain edema features from the beginning are found in traumatic brain edema caused by brain contusion, also in purulent meningitis and in meningoencephalitis.

The concomitance of mixed brain edema and meningeal inflammation and the extension method limit the variety of meningeal mixed brain edema (sometimes known as granulo-cytic brain edema).

3. Alteration of Cerebrospinal Fluid

Cerebrospinal fluid has a biomechanical role in maintaining the shape of the brain parenchima and a biochemical role in the metabolic exchanges of the nervous parenchima. CSF may interfere in the changes of the intracranial pressure by:

a. biomechanical modifications;
b. biochemical modifications.

a. Biomechanical modifications

The growth of the CSF quantity can be caused by disorders of CSF formation, circulation or resorption.

Hydrocephalus

Hydrocephalus is the abnormal accumulation of cerebrospinal fluid (CSF) in the ventricles of the brain.[4,8,9] Hydrocephalus may be congenital (present at birth) or acquired. Hydrocephalus may be communicating or non-communicating. Communicating hydrocephalus occurs when the flow of CSF is blocked after it exits the ventricles. Obstructive hydrocephalus or non-communicating hydrocephalus occurs when the flow of CSF is blocked along one or more of the narrow passages connecting the ventricles. One of the most common causes of hydrocephalus is "aqueductal stenosis." In this case, hydrocephalus results from a narrowing of the aqueduct of Sylvius, a small passage between the third and fourth ventricles in the middle of the brain. [4,12,17,20]

There are two other forms of hydrocephalus: hydrocephalus ex-vacuo and normal pressure hydrocephalus. Hydrocephalus ex-vacuo occurs when stroke or traumatic injury cause damage to the brain and brain tissue may actually shrink; the CSF pressure is normal in hydrocephalus ex-vacuo. Normal pressure hydrocephalus is most common among the elderly and may result from a subarachnoid hemorrhage, head trauma, infection etc. or for reasons that are unknown. [17,24,26,37]

The mechanisms involved in the increase of the CSF volume may be:

1. CSF hypersecretion;
2. CSF circulation disorders generated by a partial or complete obstruction of the ventricular paths or by a blocking of the peripheral CSF circulation ways, producing an obstructive hydrocephalus.
3. the diminishing of the CSF resorption that can be produced by:
   - the disorder of the membrane transfer mechanisms in the drainage venous system or by lesions of the anatomical structures that allow this transfer,
   - the increase of the intracranial venous blood pressure .
   - the passive hydrocephalus consist of the reduction of the cerebral parenchima with the passive filling of the hereby space by the CSF.

b. Biochemical changes

The modifications of the CSF chemical composition appear in various disorders:

- meningitis, encephalitis,
- brain tumors,
- arachnoiditis,
- subarachnoid hemorrhage,
- spinal cord compression etc.

In these clinical conditions, essential for the formation and the development of intracranial hypertension are only the biochemical modifications that alter the rheologic properties of CSF.

4. Cerebrovascular Reactivity

The variations of the cerebral blood volume are an instability factor for the intracranial pressure; the increase of the intracranial blood volume is frequent with important clinical manifestations.

Schematically, the ICH pathogeny by cerebral vascularization disorders can be presented in this way:

a. the affecting of the arterial blood component:
   - in the systemic high blood pressure with hydrostatic cerebral edema, when the cerebral blood flow remains constant consequently to the increase of the vascular resistance and the growth of the cerebral perfusion pressure;
   - the increase of the cerebral blood flow by the lowering of the cerebrovascular resistance in case of hypercapnia;
   - the decrease of the blood flow in the ischemic stroke and the developing of the extensive ischemic brain edema;
b. The disturbance of the venous component caused by a low venous drainage or by the blocking of the venous returning with:
   - the decrease of the CSF resorption,
   - venous stasis.

The variations that can be generated at the brain blood circulation level are generally well controlled by self-adjustment mechanisms that maintain the cerebral blood flow at normal values for blood pressures up to 160 mmHg, or in case of a patient with high blood pressure, up to 180-200 mmHg. The installation of ICH as a disease is represented by the decompensation of the ICH syndrome, when the compensatory mechanisms are exhausted and the accentuation of the endocranial volume-pressure relationship is affecting organically the brain.

From this moment the increase of the ICP has two endocranial results:

- the disorder of cerebral circulation with the affecting of the cerebral blood flow

and

- the shifting of the cerebral substance - the brain herniation between the supratentorial, subtentorial and spinal spaces, caused by the pressional gradient.

The consequences of the intracranial hypertension appear through the cerebral circulation disturbance and/or through brain herniation and are caused by ischemia, hemorrhage and direct compression of brain stem vital centers.

5. Decompensation of Intracranial Hypertension

Brain ischemia

The moderate increase of ICP does not induce marked changes in the cerebral blood flow. A bigger growth of ICP initially causes a capillary collapse and the slowing down of the blood circulation. Secondary, it generates the increase of $PaCO_2$ and the lowering of PaO_2, which determine the rise of the cerebral blood flow with vasodilatation, in spite of the increased value of ICP, therefore the cerebral perfusion pressure remains. [15,22,35]

This maintenance of the cerebral perfusion pressure involves the increase of the systolic blood pressure (the Cushing mechanism as an attempt to prevent the ischemia). Cushing described the clinical presentationof the intracranial hypertension syndrome worsening, which includes bradycardia, the increase in the systemic blood pressure, and the occurrence of respiratory disorders. These symptoms are caused by the brainstem suffering by means of a brainstem compression performed by a brain herniation or by the circulatory disorders generated by the increase in the intracranial pressure.[23,25,49]

Idiopathic intracranial hypertension has an increase in the intracranial pressure is extremely slow, with a chronic aspect. This very slow increase in the intracranial pressure allows good pressure compensation and an almost normal maintenance of the cerebral blood flux.

The good clinical condition is determined to the auto-regulation of the cerebral circulation, because the increased intracranial pressure has a reduced action on the endocranial structures in the dynamic conditions of the rapid fluid circuit. This mechanism does not occur during the other types of intracranial hypertension.

Very high increases of ICP cause the cerebral perfusion pressure to be very low, the cerebral vascular collapse and the cerebral blood flow stops. The ischemic areas exacerbate the brain edema and gradually extend themselves. [1,15,35,50]

The blocking of the cerebral circulation happens in case of a ICP value near the blood pressure (the medium value) and without pressional gradients between the dural cranio-spinal spaces. The uniform increase of ICP in endocranial compartments without the emergence of the brain herniation appears in prolonged ICH conditions with chronic character.

The period from the beginning of the cerebral circulation disorders until the stop of the cerebral blood flow varies in time and is characterized by the occurrence of ischemic lesions, initially recoverable, which then exacerbate and extend themselves, and finally affecting the diencephalon and midbrain vital centers.

The ischemia extends itself in a cranial-caudal way causing diencephalon lesions and then brain stem lesions, presenting as a gradually aggravating clinical syndrome.

It is possible that the severe neurologic syndrome during the aggravation of the chronic ICH condition is actually produced by the axial compression of the brain stem with midbrain ischemia, being therefore a mixed lesion.

Brain Herniations

Brain herniations represent shift of the normal brain through or across regions to another site due to mass effect from traumatic, neoplastic, ischemic, or infectious etiologies.[1,5,7]

Brain herniation can occur :

- between compartments inside the skull, such as those separated by a rigid membrane called the "tentorium",
- through foramen occipitalis (the natural opening at the base of the skull)
- through surgical openings created by a craniotomy procedure.

There are major types of herniation: supratentorial , infratentorial and transcalvarial herniation.

Central herniation : Central herniation, (also called "transtentorial herniation") can occur when the brain moves either up or down across the tentorium : ascending and descending transtentorial herniation ; descending herniation is much more common.The diencephalon and parts of the temporal lobes of both of the cerebral hemispheres are squeezed through a notch in the tentorium cerebella. Descending transtentorial herniations are caused by mass effect in the cerebrum which pushes the supratentorial brain to the posterior fossa. Descending transtentorial herniation includes the subcategory of uncal herniation. Uncal herniation may advance to central herniation.

Ascending transtentorial herniation or cerebellar herniation is caused by mass effect in the posterior fossa which leads to brain extending through the incisura in an upward.[1,29,36,41]

Cingulate herniation or subfalcine herniation : subfalcine herniation occurs when the supratentorial brain is displaced underneath the falx secondary to mass effect.

Alar herniation results from the supratentorial brain sliding either anteriorly or posteriorly over the wing of the sphenoid bone. There are a relative absence of clinical symptomatology.Anterior herniation is the temporal lobe herniation anteriorly and superiorly over the sphenoid bone and the posterior type is the frontal lobe herniation posteriorly and inferiorly over the sphenoid bone.

Tonsillar herniation occurs when the cerebellar tonsilsis displaced through the foramen magnum secondary to mass effect.

Transcalvarial herniation or external herniation : extracranial herniation occurs with displacement of brain through a cranial defect.[25,41,48,50]

References

[1] Adamson DC, Dimitrov DF, Bronec PR. Upward transtentorial herniation, hydrocephalus, and cerebellar edema in hypertensive encephalopathy.*Neurologist*.2005; 11(3):171-5.

[2] Adelson PD, Bratton SL, Carney NA, Chesnut RM,et al Intracranial pressure monitoring technology. *Pediatr. Crit. Care Med.* 2003 ;4(3 Suppl):S28-30

[3] Asil T, Uzunca I, Utku U, Berberoglu U. Monitoring of increased intracranial pressure resulting from cerebral edema with transcranial Doppler sonography in patients with middle cerebral artery infarction. *J. Ultrasound Med.* 2003 ;22(10):1049-53.

[4] Babapour B, Oi S, Boozari B, Tatagiba M,et al Fetal hydrocephalus, intrauterine diagnosis and therapy considerations: an experimental rat model. *Childs Nerv Syst.* 2005; 21(5):365-71

[5] Barton CW, Hemphill JC, Morabito D, Manley G. A novel method of evaluating the impact of secondary brain insults on functional outcomes in traumatic brain-injured patients. *Acad. Emerg. Med.* 2005 ;12(1):1-6.

[6] Castejon OJ. Lysosome abnormalities and lipofucsin content of nerve cells of oedematous human cerebral cortex.*J. Submicrosc. Cytol. Pathol.* 2004 ;36(3-4):263-71.

[7] Ciurea AV, Nuteanu L, Simionescu N, Georgescu S. Posterior fossa extradural hematomas in children: report of nine cases. *Childs Nerv. Syst.* 1993 ;9(4):224-8.

[8] Collmann H, Sorensen N, Krauss J. Hydrocephalus in craniosynostosis: a review.Childs Nerv Syst. 2005; 27.

[9] Czosnyka ZH, Cieslicki K, Czosnyka M, Pickard JD. Hydrocephalus shunts and waves of intracranial pressure. *Med. Biol. Eng. Comput.* 2005 ;43(1):71-7.

[10] Demchuk AM, Burgin WS, Christou I, et al. Thrombolysis in brain ischemia (TIBI) transcranial Doppler flow grades predict clinical severity, early recovery,and mortality in patients treated with intravenous tissue plasminogen activator. *Stroke.* 2001; 32: 89–93.

[11] Dickerman RD, Morgan J. Pathogenesis of subdural hematoma in healthy athletes: postexertional intracranial hypotension? Acta Neurochir (Wien). 2005;147(3):349-50..

[12] Donovan DJ. Simple depressed skull fracture causing sagittal sinus stenosis and increased intracranial pressure: case report and review of the literature.*Surg Neurol.* 2005 ;63(4):380-3.

[13] Dunn LT. Raised intracranial pressure. *J.Neurol.Neurosurg.Psychiatry*.2002;73,1:i23-7.

[14] Eide PK, Fremming AD. A computer-based method for comparisons of continuous intracranial pressure recordings within individual cases. *Acta Neurochir.* (Wien). 2003;145(5):351-7.

[15] Fischer S, Wobben M, Marti HH, Renz D, Schaper W. Hypoxia-Induced Hyperpermeability in Brain Microvessel Endothelial Cells Involves VEGF-Mediated Changes in the Expression of Zonula Occludens-1. *Microvasc. Res.* 2002 ;63(1):70-80

[16] Fischer S, Wiesnet M, Marti HH, Renz D, Schaper W. Simultaneous activation of several second messengers in hypoxia-induced hyperpermeability of brain derived endothelial cells. *J. Cell Physiol.* 2004 ;198(3):359-69.

[17] Forsyth R, Baxter P, Elliott T. Routine intracranial pressure monitoring in acute coma.*Cochrane Database Syst Rev*. 2001;(3):CD002043

[18] Fritsch MJ, Doerner L, Kienke S, Mehdorn HM. Hydrocephalus in children with posterior fossa tumors: role of endoscopic third ventriculostomy. *J. Neurosurg.* 2005 ; 103(1 Suppl):40-2

[19] Gaohua L, Kimura H. A mathematical model of intracranial pressure dynamics for brain hypothermia treatment. *J. Theor. Biol.* 2005 ; 10;

[20] Giulioni M, Ursino M. Head injury and autoregulation. J Neurosurg. 2003 ;99(2):437-8.

[21] Gjerris, F., Sarensen, P. S., Vorstrup, S., et al.: Intracranial pressure, conductance to cerebrospinal fluid outflow, and cerebral blood flow in patients with benign intracranial hypertension (pseudotumor cerebri). *Ann. Neurol.*1985 , 17:158,.

[22] Good DC, Ghobrial M: Pathologic changes associated with intracranial hypotension and meningeal enhancement on MRI. *Neurology* ,1993. 43:2698–2700,

[23] Hlatky R, Valadka AB, Robertson CS. Intracranial hypertension and cerebral ischemia after severe traumatic brain injury. *Neurosurg. Focus*. 2003 15;14(4):e2.

[24] Iencean St M Brain edema - a new classification.*Medical Hypotheses*. 2003 ;61(1):106

[25] Iencean St M Idiopathic intracranial hypertension and idiopathic normal pressure hydrocephalus: diseases with opposite pathogenesis? *Medical Hypotheses*. 2003 ;61(5-6):526-8.

[26] Iencean St M Pattern of increased intracranial pressure and classification of intracranial hypertension. *Journal of Medical Sciences*, 2004, vol.4,Nr.1 :52- 58

[27] Iencean St M Simultaneous hypersecretion of CSF and of brain interstitial fluid causes idiopathic intracranial hypertension. *Medical Hypotheses.* 2003 ;61(5-6):529-32.

[28] Jalan R. Intracranial hypertension in acute liver failure: pathophysiological basis of rational management. *Semin. Liver Dis.* 2003 ;23(3):271-82.

[29] Johnston M. The importance of lymphatics in cerebrospinal fluid transport.*Lymphat Res. Biol.* 2003;1(1):41-4.

[30] Joo F Klatzo I.Role of cerebral endothelium in brain oedema *Neurol. Res.*1989;11:67-75

[31] Katayama Y, Kawamata T. Edema fluid accumulation within necrotic brain tissue as a cause of the mass effect of cerebral contusion in head trauma patients. *Acta Neurochir. Suppl.* 2003;86:323-7

[32] Kim JH, Kim MJ, Kang JK, Lee SA. Vasogenic edema in a case of hypercalcemia-induced posterior reversible encephalopathy. *Eur. Neurol.* 2005;53(3):160-2

[33] Kurtcuoglu V, Poulikakos D, Ventikos Y. Computational modeling of the mechanical behavior of the cerebrospinal fluid system. *J. Biomech. Eng.* 2005 ;127(2):264-9.

[34] Kushi H, Saito T, Makino K, Hayashi N. Neuronal damage in pericontusional edema zone. *Acta Neurochir. Suppl.* 2003;86:339-42.

[35] Maeda T, Katayama Y, Kawamata T, Koyama S, Sasaki J. Ultra-early study of edema formation in cerebral contusion using diffusion MRI and ADC mapping. *Acta Neurochir. Suppl.* 2003;86:329-31.

[36] Marmarou A. The pathophysiology of brain edema and elevated intracranial pressure. *Cleve Clin J. Med.* 2004 ;71 Suppl 1:S6-8.

[37] Melgar MA, Rafols J, Gloss D, Diaz FG. Postischemic reperfusion: ultrastructural blood-brain barrier and hemodynamic correlative changes in an awake model of transient forebrain ischemia. *Neurosurgery.* 2005 ;56(3):571-81

[38] Mihorat TH. Classification of the cerebral edemas with references to hydrocephalus and pseudotumor cerebri . *Child Nerv. Syst* 1992;8: 301-306

[39] Mori T, Wang X, Kline AE, Siao CJ, Dixon CE, Tsirka SE, Lo EH. Reduced cortical injury and edema in tissue plasminogen activator knockout mice after brain trauma. *Neuroreport* 2001 21;12(18):4117-20

[40] Mueller E, Wietzorrek J, Ringel F, Guretzki S, Baethmann A, Plesnila N. Influence of hypothermia on cell volume and cytotoxic swelling of glial cells in vitro. *Acta Neurochir. Suppl* .2000;76:551-5

[41] Oyelese AA, Steinberg GK, Huhn SL, Wijman CA. Paradoxical cerebral herniation secondary to lumbar puncture after decompressive craniectomy for a large space-occupying hemispheric stroke: case report. *Neurosurgery.* 2005 ;57(3).

[42] Penn RD, Lee MC, Linninger AA, Miesel K, Lu SN, Stylos L. Pressure gradients in the brain in an experimental model of hydrocephalus.*J. Neurosurg.* 2005 ;102(6):1069-75.

[43] Plesnila N, Schulz J, Stoffel M, Eriskat J, Pruneau D, Baethmann A. Role of bradykinin B2 receptors in the formation of vasogenic brain edema in rats. *J. Neurotrauma* 2001 Oct;18(10):1049-58

[44] Querfurth HW, Lagreze WD, Hedges TR, Heggerick PA. Flow velocity and pulsatility of the ocular circulation in chronic intracranial hypertension. *Acta Neurol Scand.*2002 ; 105(6):431-40

[45] Rosengarten B, Ruskes D, Mendes I, Stolz E. A sudden arterial blood pressure decrease is compensated by an increase in intracranial blood volume. *J. Neurol.* 2002 ; 249(5):538-41.

[46] Stam J.Thrombosis of the cerebral veins and sinuses. *N. Engl. J. Med.* 2005, 28;352:1791-8.

[47] Suzuki R, Fukai N, Nagashijma G, et al Very early expression of vascular endothelial growth factor in brain oedema tissue associated with brain contusion. *Acta Neurochir. Suppl.* 2003;86:277-9.

[48] Schwarcz A, Berente Z, Osz E, Doczi T. In vivo water quantification in mouse brain at 9.4 Tesla in a vasogenic edema model. *Magn. Reson. Med.* 2001 Dec;46(6):1246-9.

[49] Tamburrini G, Caldarelli M, Massimi L,et al Intracranial pressure monitoring in children with single suture and complex craniosynostosis: a review.*Childs Nerv. Syst.* 2005, 3.

[50] Tamimi A, Abu-Elrub M, Shudifat A, Saleh Q, Kharazi K, Tamimi I. Superior sagittal sinus thrombosis associated with raised intracranial pressure in closed head injury with depressed skull fracture. *Pediatr. Neurosurg.* 2005 ;41(5):237-40.

[51] Wintermark M, Thiran JP, Maeder P, Schnyder P, Meuli R. Simultaneous measurement of regional cerebral blood flow by perfusion CT and stable xenon CT: a validation study. *Am. J. Neuroradiol.* 2001; 22: 905–914.

Chapter V

Clinical Presentation of Intracranial Hypertension

1. Signs and Symptoms

The symptomatology of the intracranial hypertension syndrome has been classically divided into two groups: the main signs, represented by the triad cephalea, vomiting and papillary edema, and secondary or accessory signs, which include the psychical disorders, meningeal irritation, paresis of ocular-motor nerves, vegetative disorders, sometimes comitial crises. [1,6,15,18]

It is currently believed that the combination of cephalea and eye fundus changes may be considered significant for the intracranial hypertension. The addition of psychical disorders and/or vomiting represents a pathognomic clinical picture of intracranial hypertension.

1. Cephalea

Cephalea is considered to be the most important and characteristic ICH symptom.

Cephalea is the most frequent symptom manifested in intracranial hypertension; however, it is present only in 55 - 60% of the intracranial hypertension cases in intracranial tumors, but in almost 90% of the other intracranial hypertension cases. Cephalea may be precocious, as a first symptom, with a progressive character, or it occurs later on, depending on the evolution of the illness that causes the ICH syndrome. In case of a cephalea beginning, it may persist as a single or dominant symptom for variable periods, depending on the development speed of the causal disorder. [1,3,6,7]

Depending on its location, cephalea may be generalized or diffuse, and localized.

The diffuse and permanent cephalea, with periodic exacerbations, sometimes with a pulsatile aspect and a slowly progressive accentuation (sometimes the accentuation may be faster), is considered reminiscent of the intracranial hypertension with progressive evolution. It is quite intense in the morning, due to the nocturnal increase in the intracranial pressure, and it is partially or sufficiently diminished after a vomiting episode. The usual antalgics have a limited effect. [8,9,13,14]

The identified cephalea may be permanent or intermittent, sometimes with a migraine aspect or with an unusual center and irradiation (irradiation towards the throat, the nose radix, etc.).

With a background of a permanent cephalea, the episodes of algic exacerbation may often have a localizing character, or, vice-versa, on a background of a persistent localized pain, the headache episode has the features of generalized cephalea.

Depending on the development speed of the causal disorder, and on the installation of the intracranial hypertension, cephalea generally has a progressive character, with a permanent accentuation of intensity and the increase in the frequency of the headache episodes.

In contrast to this evolutionary character of cephalea in intracranial hypertension, the cephalea manifested in other disorders maintains its characteristics for long periods.

The headache episode may occur in the morning or it may commence due to the changes in the head position: bowing, sudden rise, coughing, physical efforts, etc.

During the algic crisis, the patient finds an immobile position or he is nervous and wants to vomit, knowing that the cephalea subsequently stopped before, or he finds the most immobile position possible. Light and noise are often difficult to bear, as it happens in migraine crises.

The end of the crisis is slow, while an algic background is maintained, generally a bearable one.

At first, algic crises may be separated by long time intervals (months or weeks) and, progressively, they become more frequent and of a longer duration, with slow recovery and the persistence of a state of disorientation. [14,19,21,23]

The description of the crisis is obviously very subjective, and it depends on the presence of the simultaneous psychical disorders.

It has been noticed that cephalea diminishes or it may even disappear as the papillary edema develops into optic atrophy, without finding a convincing explanation (there is a hypothesis regarding the decrease in the cerebrospinal fluid by a concomitant atrophy at the level of the choroid plexuses).

Moreover, the intracranial hypertension in frontal tumors may not be accompanied by cephalea due to a frontal pseudo-lobotomy effect caused by the tumor.

The pathogenic mechanism that causes the cephalea has not been yet clarified; it is thought that the cephalea is caused by the increase in the intracranial pressure that produces the distension of the dura mater affecting the pain receptors.

There has been an experimental acknowledgement of the disparity between the increase in the intracranial pressure and cephalea, especially underlining the fact that the syndromes of idiopathic intracranial hypertension include very large increases in the intracranial pressure (with an important impact on the eye fundus) without cephalea or with a bearable cephalea.

The ICH cephalea is currently considered to be the result of summing several mechanisms through which the pain intracranial receptors are excited:

- cerebral venous dilatation, secondary to hypercapnia,
- traction of the cerebro-meningeal veins,
- stimulation of the nociceptors from the basal dura mater by tensioning the arteries at the skull base,

- local stimulation of the dural nociceptors in the superficial parenchymatous lesions,
- irritation and injury of certain nuclei, centers or circuits involved in the pain mechanisms, by means of the mechanical compression and structure-moving effects due to the tumor development.

Depending on the presented characteristics, there is a description of the aspects that are considered typical for the intracranial hypertension syndrome of the generalized or localized cephalea.

The generalized or diffuse cephalea has a pulsatile aspect, with a cephalic burden sensation, sometimes described as an "inside-the-hamlet" feeling, or temporally accentuated. In the case of the intracranial hypertension caused by an obstructive hydrocephalus, the cephalea is predominantly frontal or frontal-occipital, and it is worsened by physical efforts or by a change of position. [21,24,26,28]

The headache episodes are frequently connected to the movements of the head, when the circulation of the cerebrospinal fluid may be blocked.

The identified cephalea may concord with a superficial cerebral tumor location; thus the front-orbital pain may correspond to a frontal tumor; a temporal pain (sometimes accentuated at percussion) may correspond to certain temporal or Rollandic lesions, and the cerebellum tumors may be accompanied by a sub-occipital cephalea.

Depending on the patient's age and on the general clinical condition, an anamnesis may show the typical or non-characteristic aspects of cephalea.

In the case of a small child or of an infant, the agitation may suggest the manifestation of a cephalea, being necessary to correlate it with other signs and explorations.

In the case of a patient with psychic disorders, the anamnesis is difficult, and the information provided by his or her acquaintances is often irrelevant.

The cephalea alone, even with the typical aspect of intracranial hypertension, offers guidance only for the clinical examination and the paraclinical exploration.

2. Papillary Edema and Visual Disorders

Beside the cephalea the papillary edema is considered a characteristic sign because it is caused by the increase in the intracranial pressure and its evolution is in accordance with the intracranial hypertension syndrome. The installation of the papillary edema happens gradually, and there is often a correspondence with the visual acuity disorders. Thus, the anamnesis underlines the existence of several temporary loss of sight, lasting for a few seconds, which are considered as extremely suggestive for the ICH syndrome. [2,4,6,10]

The phenomenon consists in a sudden blindness, of a few seconds' duration, followed by the recovery of sight. Moreover, there is a progressive decrease in the visual acuity, as well as a diminished colour perception (the first colour that is influenced by ICH is the blue one).

The papillary edema is progressively installed, and, 1 – 2 weeks after the increase in the intracranial pressure, there is the incipient aspect of papillary contour blur, with a discrete venous dilatation, and the next step of its evolution is the manifest papillary edema, with the erasure of the papillary contour and with dilated and tortuous veins. One may notice that the optic nerve papilla disappears, it becomes turgescent, with the aspect of a venous stasis and with spastic arteries. At this stage, there may be peri-capillary hemorrhages with a typical aspect of a flame.

a

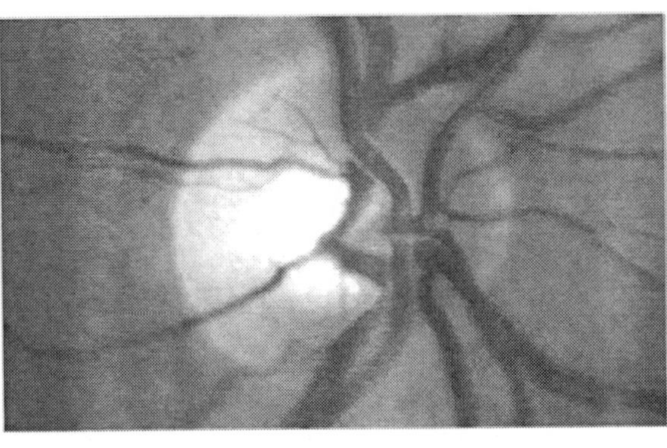

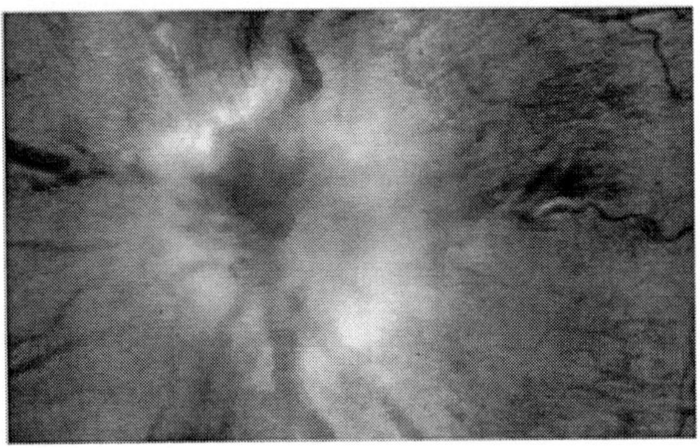

b

Figure 26. Eye fundus examination: a. normal papilla, b. papillary edema with venous stasis.

The papillary edema may be unequally developed in the two eyes, or it may be unilaterally present, perhaps in an initial relation to the location of the intracranial expansive process. [9,10,17,25]

In the case of the intracranial hypertension, there is an installation of the secondary optic atrophy. The presence of the optic atrophy corresponds to the significant diminishing of the visual acuity to blindness.

The post-stasis optic atrophy with secondary cecity represents an ophthalmoscopic aspect that is rarely present nowadays because of the increased accessibility of appropriate exploration means.

There are situations when the ICP increase is not pre-empted by the occurrence of the papillary edema:

- the acute installation of the ICH syndrome,
- a preexisting bilateral optic atrophy,
- in the case of young children, the papillary edema is rarer because the increase in the cranial volume is possible as the ICP increases.

- in the case of old people, usually after the age of 60 - 65 years old, the papillary edema is rarer or less accentuated on account of the cerebral atrophy frequency.

The pathogenic relation to the intracranial hypertension is not clear, although the ICP increase leads to the formation and the evolution of the papillary edema; according to Hayreh, 1964, the hypertension of the cerebrospinal fluid affects the optic nerve, and the stasis occurs at the level of the central retinal vein, which causes aspects of edema and papillary stasis.

In the case of the idiopathic ICH, the evolution of the papillary edema is a long one, and, sometimes, its progression towards atrophy cannot be stopped. There is a frequent decrease in the visual acuity, and, when the visual field is examined, the extension of the blind spot is underlined. A characteristic clinical aspect is often the disparity between the cephalea, which is present but minor, and the serious papillary edema that may lead to blindness. [17,27,28,30]

A particular case is the presence of the papillary edema in various stages in one eye with optic atrophy in the other. The primitive optic atrophy with central scotoma and anosmia by direct compression, and the controlateral papillary edema by intracranial hypertension constitute the Foster Kennedy syndrome, which is classically associated to frontal tumors and is especially considered pathognomic for olphactive meningiomas.

3. Vomiting

In the classical semiological presentation, vomiting is a part of the pathognomic triad for the intracranial hypertension syndrome. [4,10,17,24]

Vomiting usually occurs at a later stage in the evolution of the intracranial hypertension, and its frequency depends on the patient's age and on the cause of the ICP increase.

The clinical aspect may be as follows:

- typical for the ICH syndrome – the vomiting takes place in the morning, in jets, without nausea and without any efforts, and the cephalea calms down afterwards. Moreover, the vomiting may occur at the end of the hyper-algic cephalea episode with a moderate calming effect.
- false characteristic aspect for a digestive condition, rather frequently – with a periodicity related to meals and to the accompanying digestive symptoms,
- atypical – vomiting that has no connection to the evolution of the cephalea or to the presence of certain digestive symptoms, with varied composition (undigested, bilious, etc.) or without nausea.

The vomiting is frequently described in children with a tumor on the 4th ventricle, when it is precocious and is caused by the direct vagal irritation.

4. Psychic Disorders

Although psychic disorders are classically included in the secondary symptomatology of intracranial hypertension, they are more frequent than vomiting, which used to belong to the typical ICH syndrome. A normal psychic activity depends on a normal cerebral metabolism. The ICP increase leads to the installation and evolution of the brain edema, and to the decrease in the cerebral blood flux with a progressive diminishing of the psychic activity. [5,7,9,12,13]

At first, there is a prolonged tiresome mood with a chronic aspect, and a decline in the intellectual abilities with the background of a progressive apathy. [12,14,18]

The development also includes attention disorders, an emphasized indifference to the environment, episodes of disorientation and minor memory disorders.

The escalation of the psychic disorders corresponds to an increase in the intracranial pressure, influencing the cerebral blood flux, and it manifests itself through behaviour disorders (irritability, impulsivity, aggressiveness), impacts on the reasoning ability and a significant decrease in intellectual efficiency.

The occurrence of an intermittent somnolence mood, followed by stupor, signals the aggravation of the intracranial hypertension syndrome, with the possibility of a brain herniation, and it requires urgent measures. [12,23,28]

Besides these signs, which represent the characteristic clinical presentationof the partially compensated progressive intracranial hypertension, or before decompensation occurs, other signs may be present, too (they are less frequent and have lower significance):

- oculomotor nerves palsy with intermittent diplopia, with intermittent or permanent diplopia;
- signs of meningeal irritation (which may announce the possibility of cerebellar engagement in the absence of sub-arachnoid hemorrhage.
- endocrine disorders due to direct basal-fluid compression and to an intrasellar expansion caused by the ICH, having the secondary aspect of the Turkish saddle ("empty sella");
- convulsive crises – which are frequent in supra-tentorial tumors with intracranial hypertension; (the cortical "irritation", which is induced by the tumor, is relevant if more precociously revealed by the increase in the intracranial pressure)
- acoustic vestibular disorders – vertigoes, nistagmus, etc., which seem to depend on the tumor location in the cerebellar fosse.

The clinical presentationmay be complete or, most frequently, a certain symptom is predominant. The start may be rapid, with the manifestation of most symptoms within a short time interval, or gradual, with the slow occurrence of the symptomatology.

Depending on the patient's age, the symptomatology presents several particularities that differentiate the ICH syndrome in young children and old people from the clinical presentationof adults.

2. ICH Syndrome in Infants and Young Children

- only one symptom is often manifested: vomiting, oculomotor palsy, cephalea
- the cephalea may not always be obvious; the child is often agitated, alternating with a period of apathy, [11,16,17]
- vomiting is frequent, apparently suggesting a digestive disorder,
- one may notice the tensioning and swelling of the anterior fontanelle, or the increase in the dimensions of the skull, with suture disjunction at small children,
- at percussion, the internal hydrocephalus may be accompanied by the classical noise of an empty pot, by a "sunset" glance, and even by phenomena of epicranial venous stasis in advanced stages.
- variable changes during the eye fundus examination,
- a noisy development. [17,19,20,29]

3. ICH Syndrome in Old People

- the typical clinical signs of the intracranial hypertension are thought to occur in approximately 20 - 25% of the cases in old people.
- the clinical presentation is frequently dominated by the psychic disorders, while cephalea is non-characteristic [5,9,11]
- the eye fundus changes caused by ICH are rarer or belated,
- cardiovascular conditions, whether prior or simultaneous, make the symptom interpretation more difficult
- the intracranial hypertension symptomatology is often exceeded by the focal neurological syndrome, which is most frequently in a deficit (pareses) or irritating (convulsive crises), and which becomes dominant.

This non-characteristic symptomatology occurs in the compensated stage of the ICH syndrome with a slow evolution. [11,19,21,22]

The symptomatology is incomplete, or the relation among the existing signs is deluding, creating a false aspect that is characteristic for other conditions.

References

[1] Bergui M, Bradac GB. Clinical picture of patients with cerebral venous thrombosis and patterns of dural sinus involvement. Cerebrovasc Dis. 2003;16(3):211-6.

[2] Blaivas M, Theodoro D, Sierzenski PR. Elevated intracranial pressure detected by bedside emergency ultrasonography of the optic nerve sheath.Acad Emerg Med. 2003; 10(4):376-81.

[3] Castano A, Volcy M, Garcia FA, Uribe CS,et al Headache in symptomatic intracranial hypertension secondary to leptospirosis: a case report. Cephalalgia. 2005 ;25(4):309-11.

[4] Catz A, Reider-Groswasser I. Acoustic neurinoma and posterior fossa meningioma. Clinical and CT radiologic findings.Neuroradiology. 1986;28(1):47-52.

[5] Chambers BR, Hughes AJ. Dementia, gait disturbance, incontinence and hydrocephalus.Clin Exp Neurol. 1988;25:43-51.

[6] Chen YC, Tang LM, Chen CJ, et al. Intracranial hypertension as an initial manifestation of spinal neuroectodermal tumor. Clin Neurol Neurosurg. 2005 ;107(5):408-11

[7] Chung SJ, Kim JS, Lee MC: Syndrome of cerebral spinal fluid hypovolemia: clinical and imaging features and outcomes. Neurology 2000, 55:1321–1327.

[8] Cumurciuc R, Crassard I, Sarov M, Valade D, Bousser MG. Headache as the only neurological sign of cerebral venous thrombosis: a series of 17 cases. J Neurol Neurosurg Psychiatry. 2005; 76(8):1084-7.

[9] Dickerman RD, McConathy WJ, Lustrin E, Schneider SJ. Rapid neurological deterioration associated with minor head trauma in chronic hydrocephalus.Childs Nerv Syst. 2003 ;19(4):249

[10] Digre KB, Nakamoto BK, Warner JE et al . A comparison of idiopathic intracranial hypertension with and without papilledema. Headache. 2009 ;49(2):185-93.

[11] Drake J. Slit-ventricle syndrome. J Neurosurg. 2005 ;102(3 Suppl):257-8.

[12] Forsyth R, Baxter P, Elliott T. Routine intracranial pressure monitoring in acute coma.Cochrane Database Syst Rev. 2001;(3):CD002043..

[13] Friedman DI, Jacobson DM. Diagnostic criteria for idiopathic intracranial hypertension. Neurology. 2002 ,26;59(10):1492-5.

[14] Giulioni M, Ursino M. Head injury and autoregulation. J Neurosurg. 2003 ;99(2):437-8.

[15] Grande PO, Naredi S. Clinical studies in severe traumatic brain injury: a controversial issue. Intensive Care Med. 2002 ;28(5):529-31

[16] Hellbusch LC. Benign extracerebral fluid collections in infancy: clinical presentation and long-term follow-up. J Neurosurg. 2007 ;107(2 Suppl):119-25.

[17] Hung HL, Kao LY, Huang CC. Ophthalmic features of idiopathic intracranial hypertension. Eye. 2003 ;17(6):793-5.

[18] Kalmar AF, Van Aken J, Caemaert J, Value of Cushing reflex as warning sign for brain ischaemia during neuroendoscopy. Br J Anaesth. 2005 ;94(6):791-9.

[19] Lasjaunias P, Chiu M, ter Brugge K, et al. Neurological manifestations of intracranial dural arteriovenous malformations. J Neurosurg. 1986 ;64(5):724-30.

[20] Marcoux KK. Management of increased intracranial pressure in the critically ill child with an acute neurological injury. AACN Clin Issues. 2005 ;16(2):212-31.

[21] Norris JW, Hachinski VC. Misdiagnosis of stroke. Lancet. 1982; 1: 328–331.

[22] Reith J, Jorgensen HS, Pedersen PM, et al. Body temperature in acute stroke: relation to stroke severity, infarct size, mortality, and outcome. Lancet. 1996; 347: 422–425.

[23] Rudnick E, Sismanis A. Pulsatile tinnitus and spontaneous cerebrospinal fluid rhinorrhea: indicators of benign intracranial hypertension syndrome.Otol Neurotol. 2005 Mar;26(2):166-8.

[24] Sogawa Y, Libman R, Eviatar L, Kan L. Pulsatile Tinnitus in a 16-Year-Old Patient. Pediatr Neurol. 2005 ;33(3):214-216.

[25] Thuente DD, Buckley EG. Pediatric optic nerve sheath decompression. Ophthalmology. 2005;112(4):724-7

[26] Testa L, Mittino D, Terazzi E, Mula M, Monaco F. Cluster-like headache and idiopathic intracranial hypertension: a case report. J Headache Pain. 2008 ;9(3):181-3.

[27] van Toorn R, Georgallis P, Schoeman J. Acute cerebellitis complicated by hydrocephalus and impending cerebral herniation. J Child Neurol. 2004 ;19(11):911-3.

[28] Wall M, George D: Idiopathic intracranial hypertension. A prospective study of 50 patients. Brain, 1991, 114:155–180

[29] Weig SG. Asymptomatic idiopathic intracranial hypertension in young children. J Child Neurol. 2002 ;17(3):239-41.

[30] Wraige E, Chandler C, Pohl KR. Idiopathic intracranial hypertension: is papilloedema inevitable? Arch Dis Child. 2002 ;87(3):223-4.

Chapter VI

Decompensation of Intracranial Hypertension

1. General Data

In the case of decompensation of the intracranial hypertension syndrome, the clinical presentation changes rapidly and alarmingly:

- the typical symptoms are very accentuated: cephalea, vomiting, psychic disorders,
- the symptomatology of the causal illness may become prevailing; initial convulsive crises occur, and there is an increase in the frequency and duration of the preexisting convulsive crises, motor deficits occur or worsen; or the symptomatology of the causal illness, which is present, but discrete, becomes insignificant compared to the manifest ICH symptoms
- there are neurological and vegetative disorders, caused by the diencephalic-mesencephalic suffering, and then disorders related to the rest of the brainstem, with an aspect of a progressive worsening. [1,2,7] At the beginning of the 20th century, Cushing describes the clinical presentationof the intracranial hypertension syndrome worsening, which includes bradycardia, the increase in the systemic blood pressure, and the occurrence of respiratory disorders. These symptoms occur progressively, from the initial phase of the intracranial hypertension decompensation, and they are caused by the brainstem suffering by means of a brainstem compression performed by a brain herniation or by the circulatory disorders generated by the increase in the intracranial pressure. [8,12,29]

The neurological presentation of the ICH worsening includes:

- consciousness (vigilance) disorders: apathy, somnolence, confusion, torpor;
- coma;
- vegetative disorders (the Cushing triad),
- the pyramidal syndrome,
- injury of the cranial nerves

2. Consciousness Disorders and Coma

The neurological aggravation is announced by the occurrence or worsening of certain psychic symptoms that have diffuse effects on the vigilant state:

- a state of confusion or disorientation beside apathy, inactivity and intermittent somnolence,
- stupor and torpor – apathy, somnolence with possible motor and verbal activity;
- the state of profound somnolence, from which the patient may be awakened by verbal or algic stimulation, being able to answer questions.

These consciousness disorders (perception and vigilance) have a permanent worsening development, representing a progressive passage towards the loss of consciousness, which means a passage towards coma. [4,5,13]

Coma is already present at the moment when the symptoms of intracranial hypertension decompensation manifest themselves due to the impact on the brainstem and to the superior connections.

The worsening coma evolution through cerebral engagement is well-known, and its gravity may be periodically assessed based on the reactivity to stimulation. The depth of the coma is assessed by establishing the correlation between the intersection of the cranial nerves, the motor reaction to stimulation, and the presence of the vegetative disorders; thus the possible level of the brainstem lesion is identified. This prognosis and this assessment of the depth of the coma can be done using the Glasgow scale.

Coma symptomatology is determined by the type of brain herniation, which means it is related to the compression means that are applied to the brainstem:

- therefore, the axial brainstem herniation, with a diffuse compression, does not lead to the occurrence of a motor asymmetry,
- a unilateral temporal herniation leads to an asymmetric motor reply and the unilateral mydriasis.

Depending on the causal lesion and on the preexisting symptomatology, the clinical presentationmay be coherent by showing the accompanying neurological symptoms in accordance with the lesional or discordant level, when the neurological aspect seems imprecise.[15,17,20]

Once the coma has occurred, the prognosis depends on its profoundness, beside the etiology of the intracranial hypertension and on the type of brain herniation, which have already caused various severe lesions. The depth of the coma corresponds to the lesional level of the brainstem, and the prognosis assessment is strongly influenced by the speed of development:

- the coma installation – slowly or hurriedly
- the depth of the coma: progressive or accelerated

The typical neurological examination modifies its priorities in case of a coma, and, at the same time to the first findings, resuscitating or vital support maneuvers may be necessary (free aerial ways, cardiac frequency, efficient respiration, BP, etc.)

The evaluation of the conscience disorders, of the consciousness level, the motor reactivity and the pupil examination establish how intense and severe the existing lesions are. This assessment of consciousness-conscience modifications is based on certain scales that allow a simple and precise test.

The Glagow scale (Glasgow Coma Scale) is used, as introduced by Teasdale and Jennett in 1974:

Examination		Score
Motor response: M	Executes orders	6
	Localizes the pain	5
	Flexion on the part of the pain	4
	Abnormal flexion to pain	3
	Pathological extension	2
	Absent	1
Verbal response: V	Coherent	5
	Confuse	4
	Incoherent	3
	Unintelligible	2
	Absent	1
Ocular response: O	Spontaneous	4
	to verbal stimulus	3
	to pain	2
	Absent	1

The score represents the sum of the points for the best motor response, the best verbal response and the best ocular response; the maximum score is 15 and it corresponds to normality, while the minimum possible score is 3, and it corresponds to a state of deep coma.

The Glasgow scale evaluation expressed only by the final score may not be clear, and the Glasgow scale score must be expressed by its components.

The pediatric Glasgow scale uses the same examination adapted to the young child with reference to the specific verbal response (babbling, whining, etc.), or adapted to the preverbal stage (smile, grimaces, etc.). [1,14]

The Glasgow scale has been completed by the examination of the brainstem reflexes:

Brainstem reflexes:

- fronto-orbicular 5
- vertical oculo-vestibular 4
- papillary reflex to light 3
- horizontal oculo-vestibular 2
- oculo-cardiac 1

and this combination represents the Glasgow – Liège scale.

The use of these scales has allowed an objective and comparable assessment of patients, establishing certain therapeutic schemes for similar situations, as well as a prognosis evaluation.

3. Focal Neurological Deficit

The motor function can be affected by the initial lesion, or this can occur once the intracranial hypertension has been decompensated. [1,5,19]

The pyramidal reactivity is established in coma based on the motor response to algic stimulation and on the emphasis on the motor tonus and on reflectivity.

The motor response may be symmetrical or not in the decompensation of the intracranial hypertension syndrome, depending on the type of the primary lesion and the suffering degree of the brainstem.

The motor response may be:

- adequate towards the algic stimulation;
- aiming at the retreat of the involved limb;
- inadequate, with no finality, or extension and internal rotation for the superior limb and the extension of the inferior limb, which reveals the suffering of the brainstem.

This clinical condition corresponds to the decerebrate rigidity, which may also occur in primary lesions of the brainstem (including traumatic lesions, or in metabolic syndromes).

When the motor response is absent, the preexisting hemiparesis is accentuated, and it turns into a hemiplegia due to the compression of the brainstem at first, simultaneously with unilateral mydriasis, on the side of compression. The escalation of the engagement and the controlateral brainstem compression leads to a bi-pyramidal syndrome with bilateral mydriasis.[21,22,24,27]

The motor response allows the approximation of the axial lesion level based on the concordance of the response time, but the lesional stage assessment may also be based on the injury of the cranial nerves and on the vegetative disorders.

4. Cranial Nerve Paralysis

The first cranial nerve that is affected by the temporal cerebral herniation is the common oculomotor nerve, whose excitement is shown by the engagement ipsilateral mydriasis.

The occurrence of the unilateral mydriasis represents an alarming sign in the worsening of the clinical presentationof a supratentorial expansion. [3,16,18]

Several explanations have been suggested for the impact on the oculomotor nerve; therefore, the 3rd degree paralysis may be caused by:

- direct compression by the herniated cerebral parenchyma;
- mesencephalic ischemia – at the level of the nuclei;
- the compression of the petro-clinoidian ligament nerve;
- the compression or the traction of the nerve at the entry in the cavernous sinus;
- the compression of the oculomotor nerve at the crossing level with the posterior cerebellar artery, which is moved;
- the compression of the nerve between the posterior cerebral artery and the superior cerebellar artery.

In the late stages of the ICH decompensation, pupils become dilated and non-reactive.

The facial paralysis may be caused by a supra-nuclear lesion, and it is correlated to the preexistent pyramidal syndrome. [25,28]

The assessment of the oculo-cephalogyric and oculo-vestibular reflexes and of the deglutition reflex underlines the impact on these nerves, and it establishes the level of the lesion. This establishes how serious the brainstem suffering is, and it allows the coma prognosis to be given.

5. Vegetative Disorders

The effect of the intracranial pressure increase and of the intracranial hypertension decompression is shown by the occurrence of important cardiovascular and respiratory disorders.

Cushing's reflex is characterized by the occurrence of bradycardia, hypertension and apnea secondary to an increased intracranial pressure. [9,10]

Thus, once the intracranial pressure increase is shown to exceed the compensable values, one may notice increases in the systemic blood pressure, followed by the neurological worsening. This phenomenon has two explanations that are accepted, related to the ICH decompensation mechanisms:

- the increase in the systemic blood pressure occurs as a response to the ischemia induced by the ICP increase, and it has the role of maintaining the perfusion pressure at values that may secure a quasi-normal sanguine flow, or
- the Cushing response occurs as a vegetative disorder within the cerebral engagement with compression and brainstem suffering.

The modification of the cardiac frequency consists of bradycardia, which is obvious in the cases of ICP increase, but it is not always correlated to the variations of the blood pressure.

In the circumstances of a compensated ICH syndrome, the sudden increase in the systemic blood pressure values and the bradycardia constitute two valuable clinical signs that reveal the decompensation of the intracranial hypertension. [16,23]

In the case of a cerebral coma, regardless of its etiology, the establishment of the high blood pressureand of the bradycardia indicates the existence of an acute intracranial hypertension.

The respiratory disorders are connected to the level of the axial cerebral suffering, as there is a staged cranio-caudal deterioration in accordance with the clinical condition.

When there is a controlateral cerebral hemispheric movement, at first a diencephalic suffering is produced, and a Cheyne – Stokes respiration may also occur.

The continued ICP increase and the cerebral hernia with the brainstem hernia cause Cheyne - Stokes respiratory disorders, or a neurogenic hyper-ventilation occurs in the mesencephalic compression, while the superior compression of brainstem is accompanied by the apneusis respiration.

The coma escalation with the aggravation of the brainstem suffering by the inferior extension of the lesions that are secondary to the brain herniation compression, cause the occurrence of a superficial and rapid, inefficient breathing, and the end corresponds to an irregular, ataxic breathing.

Beside these respiratory rhythm disorders, which are always present based on the degree and level of the impact on the brainstem, a relatively rarer disorder is also described, and it is represented by the neurogenic pulmonary edema.

The intracranial hypertension can cause the neurogenic pulmonary edema based on the suffering of the hypothalamus, of the spinal bulb or of the cervical spinal marrow, and the pulmonary edema could be induced by a sympathetic stimulation with a massive adrenergic discharge, though with no possibility of establishing the formation mechanism.

The above-mentioned symptoms are associated, depending on the lesions produced by the decompensation of the intracranial hypertension, leading to characteristic clinical presentations. [23,25,27]

6. Decompensated Intracranial Hypertension

The clinical presentation of progressive aggravation through axial ischemic lesions of the diencephalon and of the brainstem is superposed and can coincide with the clinical aspects determined by the brainstem axial herniation (trans-tentorial central herniation).[6,8,11]

In the diencephalic ischemic lesion or in the general controlateral cerebral hemispheric movement, with a diencephalic compression, the clinical presentationincludes:

- moderated or accentuated somnolence (stupor);
- the preexistent pyramidal syndrome remains stationary;
- the pupil reactivity is normal;
- intermittent Cheyne - Stokes respiratory disorders may occur

The mesencephalic ischemic injury by various impacts on the cerebral circulation or by a direct brain herniation compression leads to:

- coma;
- the moments of aggravation of the preexistent neurological symptoms are preceded or accompanied by vegetative disorders: tensional oscillations (Cushing phenomenon), bradycardia, neurogenic pulmonary edema.
- the preexistent unilateral pyramidal syndrome can escalate and it rapidly turns into a bipyramidal syndrome, while the motor reactivity to the algic stimulation is of a unilateral or bilateral extension;
- the pupil reactivity diminishes;
- the Cheyne - Stokes type breathing or the neurogenic hyper-ventilation.

The caudal extension of the ischemic and compressive lesions is accompanied by the aggravation of the clinical presentation with serious brainstem suffering: deep coma with bilateral motor response in extension, pupil non-reactivity, superficial and irregular breathing. [11,17,20]

In the case of the unilateral temporal herniation, the aggravation staging is similar, with the difference represented by the existence and the escalation of the focal syndrome.

Thus, in the initial brain herniation stage, the clinical presentation includes:

- confusion syndrome, agitation or somnolence;
- cephalea and vomiting are worsening;
- the unilateral pyramidal syndrome is aggravated;
- the unilateral common oculomotor paralysis occurs, with unilateral mydriasis, non-reactive to light.
- hyperpnea respiratory disorders may occur.

The continuation of the compression on the mesencephalon manifests itself by:

- coma status;
- a bilateral pyramidal syndrome occurs with motor response to pain, initially in flexion, then in extension, unilateral and then bilateral;
- bilateral mydriasis, non-reactive to light;
- deglutition disorders;
- respiratory disorders (the Cheyne – Stokes type);
- possibly bradycardia.

Afterwards, the evolution is the same as in the case of central cerebral herniation with serious lesions of brainstem.

The herniation of the cerebellar amygdales in moderate engagements leads to nape stiffness, cephalea and aggravated vomiting, minor deglutition disorders; and, in the case of an accentuated engagement:

- hyper-extension of the neck;
- significant deglutition disorders;
- vegetative disorders;

- coma status;
- bilateral mydriasis.

The severe clinical presentation of the decompensated intracranial hypertension often illustrates the irreversibility of the ischemic and hemorrhagic lesions, which happen at the level of the vital encephalic structures. [17,26]

References

[1] Adams HP Jr, Brott TG, Crowell RM, et al. Guidelines for the management of patients with acute ischemic stroke: a statement for healthcare professionals from a special writing group of the Stroke Council, American Heart Association. *Circulation.* 1994; 90: 1588–1601.

[2] Adamson DC, Dimitrov DF, Bronec PR. Upward transtentorial herniation, hydrocephalus, and cerebellar edema in hypertensive encephalopathy. *Neurologist.* 2005; 11(3):171-5.

[3] Albayram S, Wasserman BA, Yousem DM, et al: Intracranial hypotension as a cause of radiculopathy from cervical epidural venous engorgement: case report. *AJNR,* 2002,23:618–621

[4] Alp H, Tan H, Orbak Z, Keskin H. Acute hydrocephalus caused by mumps meningoencephalitis. *Pediatr. Infect. Dis. J.* 2005 ;24(7):657-8.

[5] Barbagallo GM, Platania N, Schonauer C. Long-term resolution of acute, obstructive, triventricular hydrocephalus by endoscopic removal of a third ventricular hematoma without third ventriculostomy. Case report and review of the literature. *J. Neurosurg.* 2005;102(5):930-4.

[6] Brandt T, Pessin MS, Kwan ES, Caplan LR. Survival with basilar artery occlusion. *Cerebrovasc. Dis.* 1995; 5: 182–187.

[7] Chamberlain CE, Fitzgibbon E et al Idiopathic intracranial hypertension following kidney transplantation: A case report and review of the literature. *Pediatr. Transplant.* 2005 ; 9 (4):545.

[8] Coppage KH, Sibai BM. Treatment of hypertensive complications in pregnancy. *Curr. Pharm. Des.* 2005;11(6):749-57.

[9] De Simone R, Marano E, Fiorillo C et al Sudden re-opening of collapsed transverse sinuses and longstanding clinical remission after a single lumbar puncture in a case of idiopathic intracranial hypertension. Pathogenetic implications. *Neurol. Sci.* 2005 Feb;25(6):342-4.

[10] Dickerman RD, McConathy WJ, Lustrin E, Schneider SJ. Rapid neurological deterioration associated with minor head trauma in chronic hydrocephalus.*Childs Nerv. Syst.* 2003 ;19(4):249

[11] Donnan GA, Davis SM. Surgical decompression for malignant middle cerebral artery infarction: a challenge to conventional thinking. *Stroke.* 2003 ;34(9):2307.

[12] Ferro JM, Lopes MG, Rosas MJ, et al Delay in hospital admission of patients with cerebral vein and dural sinus thrombosis. *Cerebrovasc. Dis.* 2005;19(3):152-6.

[13] Fuentes S, Métellus P, Adetchessi T, Dufour H, Grisoli F. Hydrocefalie aigue obstructive idiopathique. A propos d'un cas.. Neurochirurgie. (fr) 2006;52(1):47-51.

[14] Fraser JF, Hartl R. Decompressive craniectomy as a therapeutic option in the treatment of hemispheric stroke. *Curr. Atheroscler. Rep.* 2005 ;7(4):296-304.

[15] Hlincik P, Nowitzke A. Rapid fluctuations in conscious state in a patient with an extensive spinal dural fistula. *J. Clin. Neurosci.* 2005 ;12(6):717-20.

[16] Iencean St M Classification and essential conditions of decompensation in intracranial hypertension ,*Rom J. Neurosurgery* 2004,Vol. I No. 1, pp. 3-13

[17] Inenaga C, Tanaka T, Sakai N, et al: Diagnostic and surgical strategies for intractable spontaneous intracranial hypotension. Case report. *J. Neurosurg.* 94:642–645, 2001

[18] Kanazawa M, Sanpei K, Kasuga K. Recurrent hypertensive brainstem encephalopathy.*J. Neurol. Neurosurg. Psychiatry.* 2005 ;76(6):888-90.

[19] Kontopoulos V, Foroglou N, Patsalas J, et al Decompressive craniectomy for the management of patients with refractory hypertension: should it be reconsidered? *Acta Neurochir.* (Wien).2002; 144(8):791-6.

[20] Kremer S, Taillandier L, Schmitt E, Bologna S, Moret C, Picard L, Bracard S. Atypical clinical presentation of intracranial hypotension: coma. *J. Neurol.* 2005 ,18

[21] Lam WW, Leung TW, Chu WC, Yeung DT,et al Early computed tomography features in extensive middle cerebral artery territory infarct: prediction of survival. *J. Neurol. Neurosurg. Psychiatry.* 2005 ;76(3):354-7.

[22] Linskey ME, Sekhar LN, Hecht ST. Emergency embolectomy for embolic occlusion of the middle cerebral artery after internal carotid artery balloon test occlusion: case report. *J. Neurosurg.* 1992; 77: 134–138.

[23] Oyelese AA, Steinberg GK, Huhn SL, Wijman CA. Paradoxical cerebral herniation secondary to lumbar puncture after decompressive craniectomy for a large space-occupying hemispheric stroke: case report. *Neurosurgery.* 2005 ;57(3)

[24] Santarius T, Menon DK. Images in clinical medicine. Carotid-artery thrombosis secondary to basal skull fracture. *N. Engl. J. Med.* 2003 , 31;349(5):e5.

[25] Shetty T. Ocular flutter in a patient with intracranial hypertension following cerebral venous thrombosis *Neurology.* 2003 11;60(3):525.

[26] Soffietti R, Ruda R, Mutani R. Management of brain metastases.*J. Neurol.*2002; 249(10):1357

[27] Stanley TV. Idiopathic intracranial hypertension presenting as hemiplegic migraine. *Acta Paediatr.* 2002;91(8):980-2.

[28] Thuente DD, Buckley EG. Pediatric optic nerve sheath decompression. *Ophthalmology.* 2005;112(4):724-7

[29] Woodworth GF, McGirt MJ, Williams MA, Rigamonti D. The use of ventriculoperitoneal shunts for uncontrollable intracranial hypertension without ventriculomegally secondary to HIV-associated cryptococcal meningitis. *Surg. Neurol.* 2005 ;63(6):529-31

Chapter VII

Paraclinical Explorations

1. General Data

The paraclinical diagnosis in neurology and neurosurgery improved continuously at the end of the 20th century through the development of investigation means that allow a precocious and highly accurate diagnosis of the cranial-cerebral lesions.

The paraclinical explorations in intracranial hypertension are based on the anamnesis and the clinical presentation, depending though on the clinical stage of the intracranial hypertension.

In the case of a hypothetic ICH syndrome, with a clinical presentation that has a slow development with non-characteristic cephalea, without a clear neurological syndrome:

- the eye fundus is examined during a complete ophthalmologic examination,
- the cranial-cervical radiographic exploration is performed, and then
- the computer tomography cerebral exploration is done.
- if the patient manifests anamnestic convulsive crises, the electroencephalographic exploration is also performed, which may reveal a lesional focus.

As the cerebral hemispheric lesions, which are slowly expansive, may often generate insignificant EEG changes, and the subtentorial lesions do not produce EEG abnormalities, this exploration does not provide useful information for the ICH diagnosis. [1,2,3,19]

The obvious ICH syndrome, with an eloquent chart and with characteristic symptoms (cephalea, nausea, vomiting, initially minor psychic disorders – apathy, adynamia, confusion, etc.):

- the ophthalmologic examination is performed, as well as
- the cranio-cerebral computer tomography exploration; then, if necessary, the MRI cerebral exploration is also performed.

Suspicion of a decompensated intracranial hypertension: in the case of a patient with a critical condition or who is in a coma (serious condition), when the anamnesis and the neurological examination emphasize the suspicion of a cerebral lesion, the exploration using the computer cranial-cerebral tomography or the cerebral nuclear magnetic resonance is urgently performed (as well as a cranial and cervical radiography in traumatisms).

The ultrasound scan performed during a pregnancy may reveal the existence of a hydrocephalus in the fetus; moreover, the cranial-cerebral ultrasound in new-born babies and infants brings clues related to the infant's hydrocephalus.

2. The Ophthalmologic Examination

The ophthalmologic examination includes the eye fundus, the testing of the visual acuity and of the visual field performed by the ophthalmologist. [9,15,19]

The eye fundus examination included in the neurological examination must be repeated and confirmed by the ophthalmologist, who can differentiate between the papillary edema at various stages and the papillary stasis and other retina modifications (papillitis, etc.).

The papilledema is a delayed consequence of the chronic CSF accumulation in the retro-bulbar optic nerve dural sheath due to the raised intracranial pressure.

The papillary edema occurs gradually: the incipient blurring aspect of the papillary contour with a direct venous dilatation is obvious 1 – 2 weeks after the increase in the intracranial pressure; the manifest papillary edema consists of the erasure of the papillary contour with dilated and tortuous veins, accompanied by the erasure of the margins of the optic nerve papilla, which becomes turgescent, with an aspect of venous stasis and with spastic arteries. At this stage, there may be pericapillary hemorrhages with the characteristic aspect of a flame.

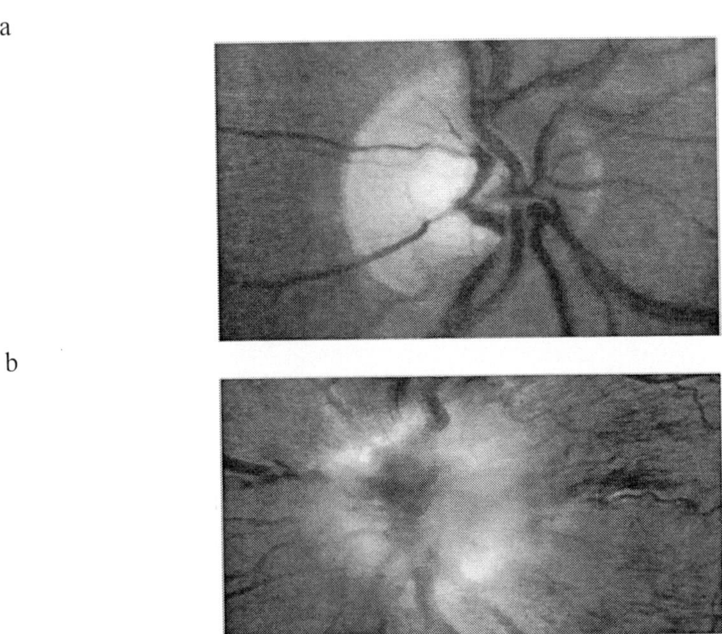

Figure 26. Eye fundus examination: a. normal papilla, b. papillary edema with venous stasis

The papillary edema can be unequal in the two eyes, or it may be unilaterally present, depending initially on the location of the expansive intracranial process.

The secondary optic atrophy occurs in prolonged, partially compensated ICH cases, and it consists of papillary excavation, with the reoccurrence of the papilla margin delimitation, and it corresponds to a diminished visual acuity to cecity. [31,34]

There are variations related to the etiopathogeny of the intracranial hypertension, age, etc.: the papillary edema is rarer in young children because, as the intracranial pressure increases, the cranial volume may increase, too; or, in old people, usually over 65 years of age, the papillary edema is rarer or less severe due to the frequency of the cerebral atrophy.

3.Skull X-Ray

The cranial radiographic exploration provides few elements for the diagnosis of the intracranial hypertension syndrome, and it is usually irrelevant from an etiological point of view. The simple cranium radiography currently has a reduced and almost historic value in the exploration of the intracranial hypertension. [4,15,17,19]

The most frequent radiographic signs that can be visible on the cranial radiography, after a long evolution of intracranial hypertension, are the following ones:

- suture dehiscence,
- sellar modification – widening of the Turkish saddle in omega; the sellar dorsum and the sellar plate grow thinner, there is a depression of the sellar tubercle, and a descent of the sphenoid plane,
- general decalcification of the skull-.

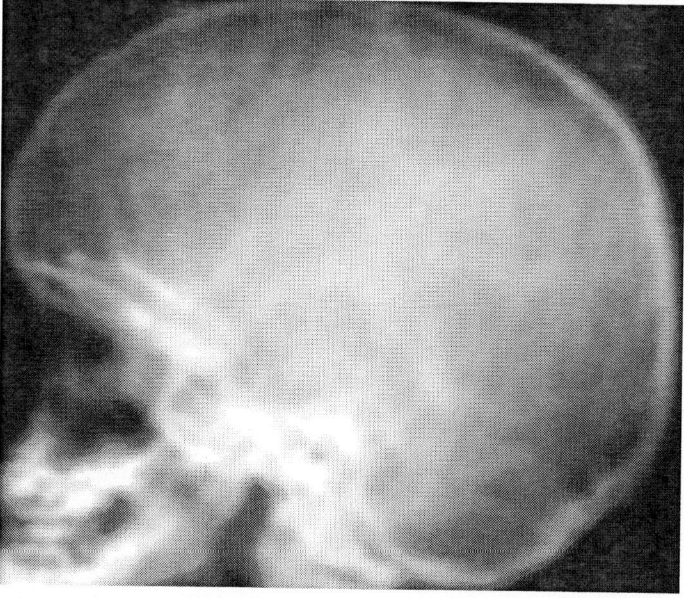

Figure 27. Child profile cranial radiography in intracranial hypertension.

The cranial radiographic modifications, which are caused by the intracranial hypertension, occur after a development of more than 2 months, and they are more obvious in children, when they occur at the level of the skull (suture disjunction etc.). In the case of adults and old people suffering from an ICH syndrome with a long development, bone modifications are visible at the level of the skull base, especially at the sellar level. [23,28,31,32]

4. CT Scan

In the case of an intracranial hypertension syndrome, the first exploration that is usually performed is the CT scan, both in neurological or neurosurgical emergencies, and in sub-acute or chronic ICH syndromes. [3,6,8,12]

The cerebral computer tomography may reveal the presence of:

- an intracranial space-replacing lesion: tumor, hematic collection, etc., identifying the location, dimensions, and the relationships with the neighbouring structures
- the brain edema, its location and extension,
- movement of the median line, the presence of a cerebral hernia,
- the presence, compression or absence of the basal cisterns,
- the presence of the hydrocephalus, etc.
- the presence of traumatic bone lesions, or of lesions that are secondary to other disorders, especially at the level of the skull base.

The use of intravenously injected contrast substances may show the increased contrast on the CT scan images at the level of a parenchymatous or perilesional lesion due to:

- the increased cerebral capillary permeability or the injury of the capillary endothelial integrity, or
- the extension of the vascular bed with a capillary permeability modified in:
- the peritumoral hyper-vascularization because of the new vessels whose endothelium lacks occlusion junctions, which are characteristic to a normal cerebral capillary;
- a decreased vascular auto-regulation in traumatic brain injury or in subintrant crises of epilepsy,
- the hyperemia from the inflammatory lesions.

In the case of the intracranial hypertension syndrome, the CT scan shows:

- the change of the gyral grooves,
- the size of the lateral ventricles:
- the lateral ventricles may be collapsed or absent in a generalized brain edema, etc.,
- the ventricular system may be dilated in the blocked circulation of the cerebrospinal fluid due to various reasons,
- the distinction between the gray matter and the white matter disappears;

- the compression or obliteration of the suprasellar cistern;
- the compression or obliteration of the quadrigeminal cistern

or it certifies a cerebral hernia:

- sub-falciform herniation or the supra-tentorial median movement,
- trans-tentorial herniation or temporal herniation,
- central herniation or trans-tentorial herniation of the brainstem,
- the subtentorial or cerebellum herniations: inferior herniation of cerebellum amygdales or superior herniation of vermis. [13,`5,17,18,22,24,25,31]

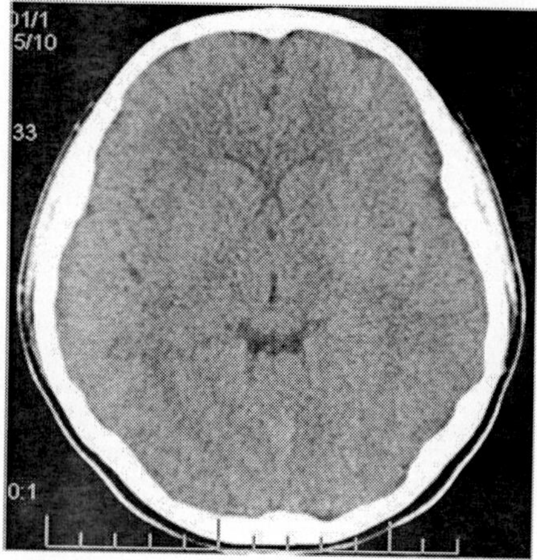

Figure 28. Generalized brain edema with the obliteration of the epicerebral space and with collapsed lateral ventricles on the CT scan image in an acute ICH syndrome .

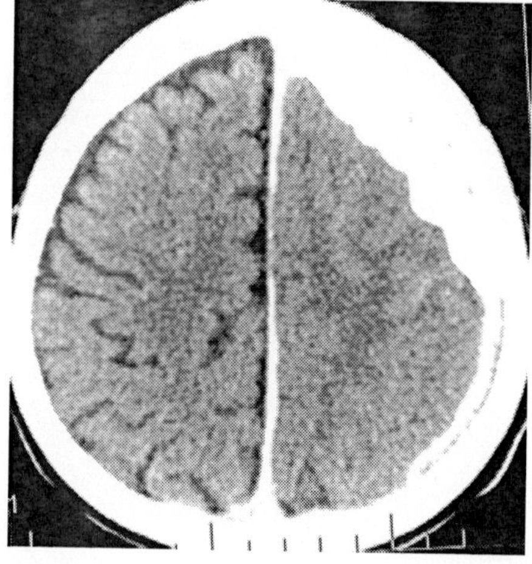

Figure 29. Left frontal subdural hematoma with left unilateral brain edema. The distinction between the white matter and the gray one is maintained, and the gyral grooves are visible in the cerebral hemisphere, controlateral to the hematoma

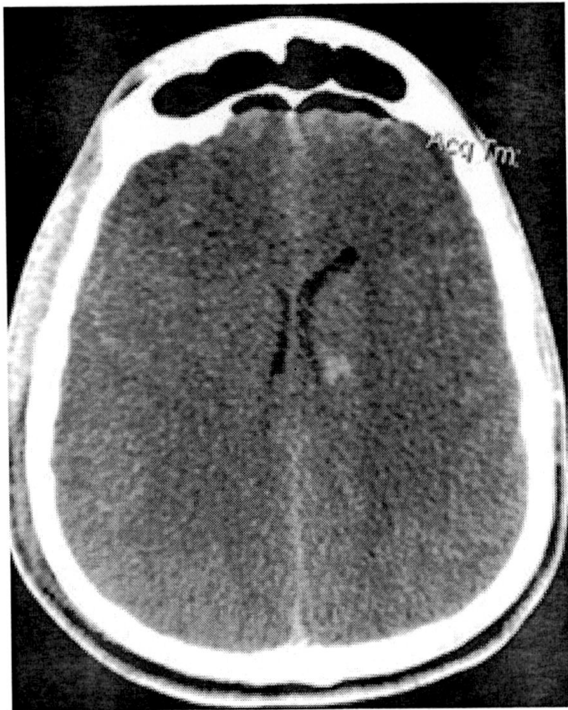

Figure 30. Traumatic brain edema with the without distinction between the gray matter and the white matter and the collapse of the lateral ventricles.

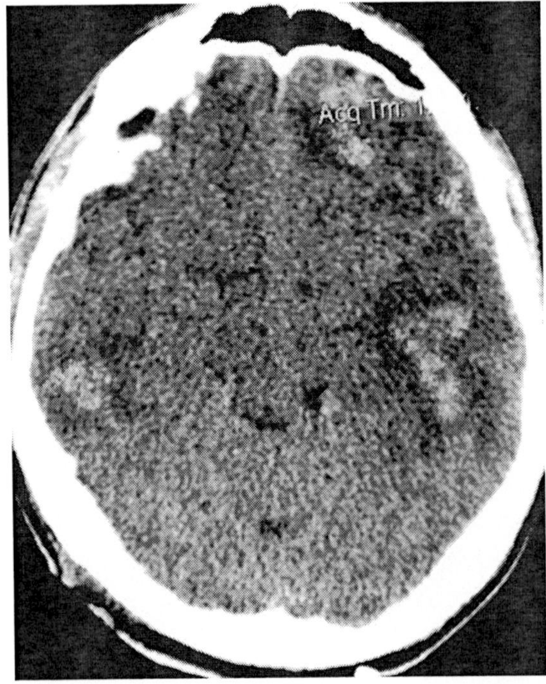

Figure 31. Multiple cerebral contusions with perilesional edema and collapse of the ventricular system .

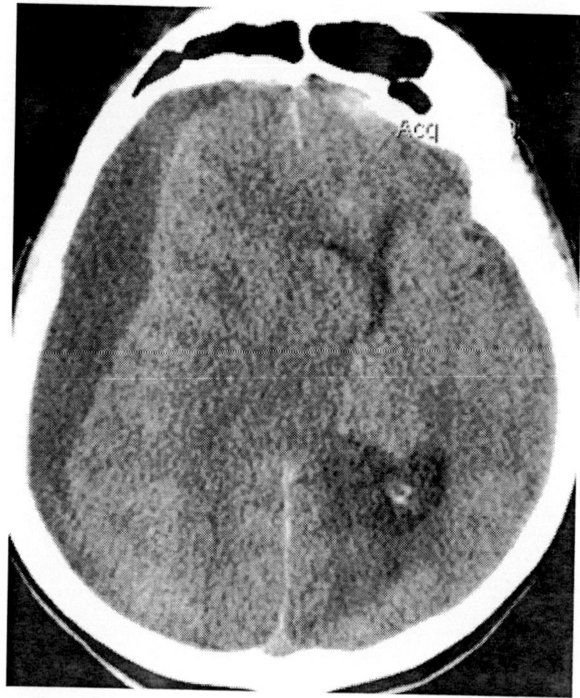

Figure 32. Subdural hematoma with sub-falciform herniation,

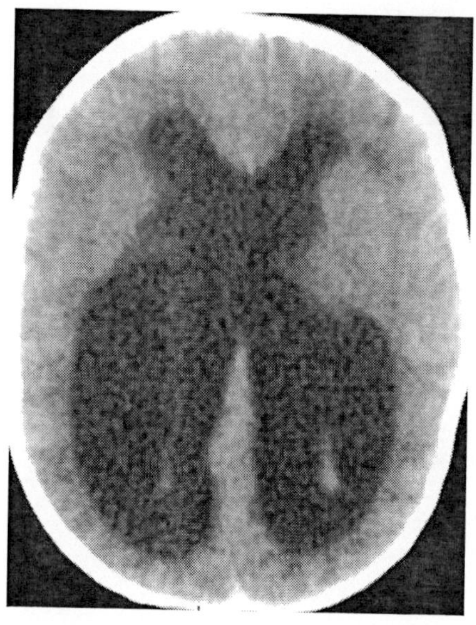

Figure 33. Internal hydrocephalus

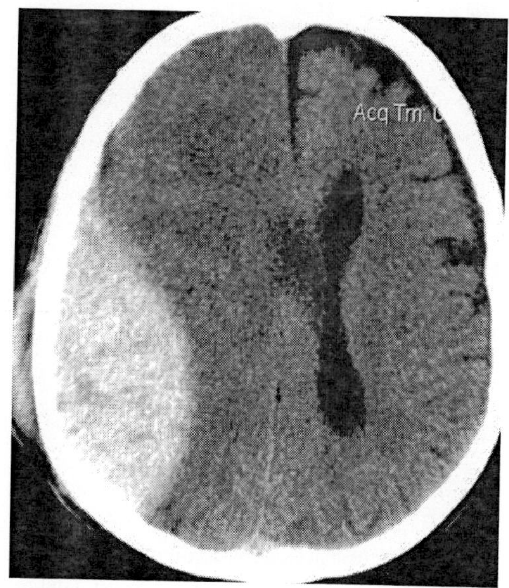

Figure 34. Extradural hematoma with compression and movement of the ventricular system to the left.

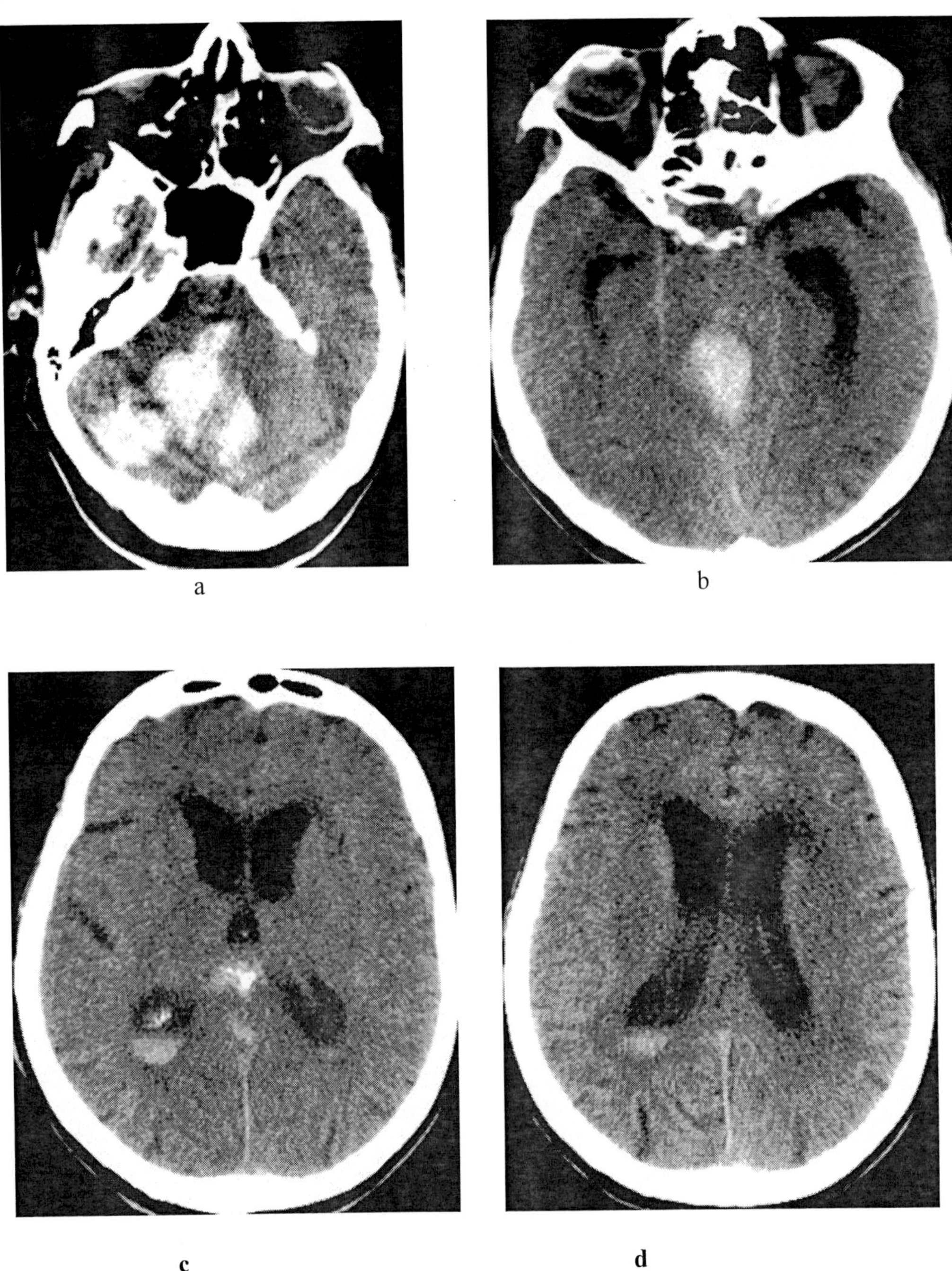

Figure 35. Cerebellum hematoma (a) with hemorrhage in the 4th ventricle (b) and with secondary acute hydrocephalus (c, d); clinically – acute ICH syndrome .

5. Magnetic Resonance Imaging (MRI).

The cerebral computer tomography allows the rapid exploration of the nervous system condition; it is extremely useful in emergencies, and it is more specific than MRI for the outlining of the acute hemorrhage. CT scan identifies the presence of the intracranial expansive process, of the brain edema, as well as the impact on the neighbouring structures. In case of traumatic emergencies, CT establishes the presence of the expansive surgical lesions, and it also allows the differentiation between the ischemic or hemorrhagic ictal lesions. [2,15,16]

The nuclear magnetic resonance is less used in the case of patients who are in coma (mainly because of the intensive therapy devices). It is very useful for the exploration of the expansive lesions from the posterior fosse and for the outlining of the arterial-venous malformations. It is superior to the computer tomography in relation to the intrinsic lesions of the cerebral substance.

The nuclear magnetic resonance shows the brain edema, and the magnetic resonance of diffusion and perfusion can differentiate the cellular edema (cytotoxic) from the extracellular brain edema (induced by oncotic-vasogenic means). Moreover, the MRI exploration shows quite well the ischemic brain edema and very well the intracellular hydrocephalic brain edema.

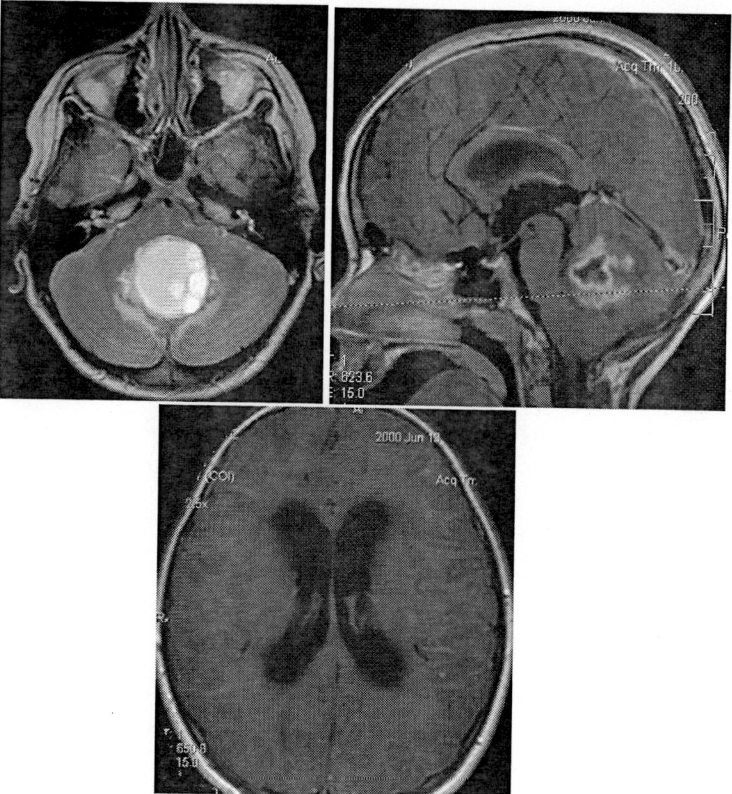

Figure 36. Cerebellar tumor and blocked fourth ventricle, secondary obstructive hydrocephalus and intracranial hypertension.

MRI can be used to measure the intracranial pressure based on the diameter of optic nerve and its sheath [optic nerve sheath diameter = ONSD]. Optic nerve sheath diameter can be measured on T2-weighted turbo spin-echo fat-suppressed sequence MRI. Measurement of ONSD is possible in 95% of cases. The ONSD is greater in TBI patients with raised ICP (>20 mmHg) than in those with ICP $\leq$ 20 mmHg, and enlarged ONSD is a predictor of raised ICP: an optic nerve sheath diameter above 5.82 mm is associated to a 90% probability of raised ICP. [20,21,27]

6. Intracranial Pressure Measurement

The intracranial pressure measurement is the exploration that reveals the ICP increase, and which directly confirms the intracranial hypertension syndrome. The clinical presentation shows the consequences of the intracranial hypertension, and the paraclinical explorations show the changes brought about by ICH. [1,5,7,10,14]

The methods used for the ICP measurement are described in the chapter on intracranial pressure. The calculation of the intracranial pressure and its monitoring allow the surveillance of pressure variations, the calculation of the cerebral perfusion pressure, the outlining of the resorption capacity of the cerebrospinal fluid, and the assessment of the intracranial compensation capacities.

The medical treatment is performed based on these parameters, assessing the occurrence of any event that may impose the repetition of the cranial-cerebral computer tomography exploration in order to identify any surgical complication. [14,15,16,26]

The indications related to the intracranial pressure monitoring concern all the cases of severe traumatic brain injury, but ICP may also be monitored in cases of idiopathic intracranial hydrocephalus, in cases of fulminating hepatic insufficiency with ICP increase, etc.

The ICP monitoring allows the assessment of modified cerebral-vascular reactivity.

The dynamic relationship between intracranial pressure and cerebral perfusion pressure is expressed by the pressure-reactivity index = PRx .

The changes in arterial blood pressure produce changes in cerebral blood volume and in intracranial pressure. But the changes in arterial blood pressure are passively transmitted to intracranial pressure when the cerebral-vascular reactivity is disturbed.

The pressure-reactivity index is determined by calculating the correlation coefficient among 40 consecutive, time-averaged data points of ICP and ABP. [11]

A normal reactivity corresponds to a negative value of PRx, while a positive value of PRx corresponds to a non-reactive cerebral-vascular bed and it indicates a poor auto-regulation and disturbed ICP reactivity. Therefore continuous monitoring with the PRx may guide the treatment of patients by identifying the optimal CPP for pressure-reactivity. [11]

The ICP modification can be important in fulminating hepatic insufficiency because it precociously shows the ICP increase and it supplies very important data concerning the possibility of neurological recovery, even in the case of a low cerebral perfusion pressure, in view of a hepatic transplant. The ICP monitoring must be considered in the case of mechanically ventilated patients, with 3rd or 4th degree encephalopathy, with a bad prognosis, but who fulfill the conditions for a hepatic transplant. [28,29,30,33]

Detailed supplementary data on ICP monitoring and on the stages of the intracranial pressure monitoring are included in the chapter about the acute intracranial hypertension in traumatic brain injury.

References

[1] Adelson PD, Bratton SL, Carney NA, Chesnut RM,et al Intracranial pressure monitoring technology. *Pediatr. Crit. Care Med.* 2003 ;4(3 Suppl):S28-30.

[2] Akbar M, Stippich C, Aschoff A. Magnetic resonance imaging and cerebrospinal fluid shunt valves. *N. Engl. J. Med.* 2005 Sep 29;353(13):1413-4.

[3] Ali SA, Cesani F, Zuckermann JA, et al: Spinal-cerebrospinal fluid leak demonstrated by radiopharmaceutical cisternography. *Clin. Nucl. Med.* 1998, 23:152–155

[4] Alvarez-Linera J, Escribano J, Benito-Leon J, et al: Pituitary enlargement in patients with intracranial hypotension syndrome. *Neurology* 2000, 55:1895–1897,

[5] Asil T, Uzunca I, Utku U, Berberoglu U. Monitoring of increased intracranial pressure resulting from cerebral edema with transcranial Doppler sonography in patients with middle cerebral artery infarction. *J. Ultrasound Med.* 2003 ;22(10):1049-53.

[6] Babapour B, Oi S, Boozari B, Tatagiba M,et al Fetal hydrocephalus, intrauterine diagnosis and therapy considerations: an experimental rat model. *Childs Nerv. Syst.* 2005;21(5):365-71.

[7] Balestreri M, Czosnyka M, Steiner LA, et al Intracranial hypertension: what additional information can be derived from ICP waveform after head injury? *Acta Neurochir.* (Wien). 2004 146(2):131-41

[8] Benamor M, Tainturier C, Graveleau P, et al: Radionuclide cisternography in spontaneous intracranial hypotension. *Clin. Nucl Med.*,1998, 23:150–151

[9] Blaivas M, Theodoro D, Sierzenski PR. Elevated intracranial pressure detected by bedside emergency ultrasonography of the optic nerve sheath.*Acad. Emerg. Med.* 2003; 10(4):376-81.

[10] Chen CC, Luo CL, Wang SJ, et al: Colour Doppler imaging for diagnosis of intracranial hypotension. *Lancet* 1999, 354:826–829,

[11] Czosnyka M, Smielewski P, Timofeev I, Lavinio A, Guazzo E, Hutchinson P, Pickard JD.Intracranial Pressure: More Than a Number, *Neurosurg. Focus* , 2007,22 (5):E10,

[12] Drake J. Slit-ventricle syndrome. *J. Neurosurg.* 2005 Apr;102(3 Suppl):257-8.

[13] Eide PK. The relationship between intracranial pressure and size of cerebral ventricles assessed by computed tomography.*Acta Neurochir* (Wien). 2003 ;145(3):171-9;

[14] Forsyth R, Baxter P, Elliott T. Routine intracranial pressure monitoring in acute coma.*Cochrane Database Syst Rev.* 2001;(3):CD002043

[15] Friedman DI, Jacobson DM. Diagnostic criteria for idiopathic intracranial hypertension. *Neurology.* 2002 26;59(10):1492-5.

[16] Gjerris, F., Sarensen, P. S., Vorstrup, S., et al.: Intracranial pressure, conductance to cerebrospinal fluid outflow, and cerebral blood flow in patients with benign intracranial hypertension (pseudotumor cerebri). *Ann. Neurol.*, 17:158, 1985.

[17] Hlatky R, Valadka AB, Robertson CS. Intracranial hypertension and cerebral ischemia after severe traumatic brain injury. *Neurosurg Focus.* 2003 15;14(4):e2.

[18] Hung HL, Kao LY, Huang CC. Ophthalmic features of idiopathic intracranial hypertension. *Eye.* 2003 ;17(6):793-5.

[19] Iencean St M Simultaneous hypersecretion of CSF and of brain interstitial fluid causes idiopathic intracranial hypertension. *Medical Hypotheses.* 2003 ;61(5-6):529-32.

[20] Kalafut MA, Schriger DL, Saver JL, Starkman S. Detection of early CT signs of >1/3 middle cerebral artery infarctions: interrater reliability and sensitivity of CT interpretation by physicians involved in acute stroke care. *Stroke.* 2000; 31: 1667–1671.

[21] Kidwell CS, Alger JR, Gobin YP, Sayre J et al MR signatures of infarction vs. salvageable penumbra in acute human stroke: a preliminary model. *Stroke.* 2000; 31: 285.

[22] Kidwell CS, Saver JL, Mattiello J, et al. A diffusion-perfusion MRI signature predicting hemorrhagic transformation following intra-arterial thrombolysis. *Stroke.* 2001; 58: 587–593.

[23] Koss SA, Ulmer JL, Hacein-Bey L: Angiographic features of spontaneous intracranial hypotension. *AJNR*, 2003, 24:704–706

[24] von Kummer R, Nolte PN, Schnittger H, Thron A, Ringelstein EB. Detectability of cerebral hemisphere ischaemic infarcts by CT within 6 h of stroke. *Neuroradiology.* 1996; 38: 31–33.

[25] Lam WW, Leung TW, Chu WC, Yeung DT,et al Early computed tomography features in extensive middle cerebral artery territory infarct: prediction of survival. *J. Neurol. Neurosurg Psychiatry.* 2005 ;76(3):354-7.

[26] Marcoux KK. Management of increased intracranial pressure in the critically ill child with an acute neurological injury. *AACN Clin Issues.* 2005 ;16(2):212-31.

[27] O'Connor W, Silberstein SD. MRI of a brain under pressure.*Headache* 2005;45(1):68-9.

[28] Penn RD, Lee MC, Linninger AA, Miesel K, Lu SN, Stylos L. Pressure gradients in the brain in an experimental model of hydrocephalus.*J. Neurosurg.* 2005 ;102(6):1069-75.

[29] Piper I, Barnes A, Smith D, Dunn L. The Camino intracranial pressure sensor: is it optimal technology? An internal audit with a review of current intracranial pressure monitoring technologies.*Neurosurgery.* 2001 ;49(5):1158-64.

[30] Quattrone A, Bono F, Pardatscher K. Manometry combined with cervical puncture in idiopathic intracranial hypertension.*Neurology.* 2002 24;59(6):963.

[31] Rudy C. Hydrocephalus. J Pediatr Health Care. 2005 ;19(2):111, 127-8.

[32] Santarius T, Menon DK. Images in clinical medicine. Carotid-artery thrombosis secondary to basal skull fracture. *N. Engl. J. Med.* 2003 , 31;349(5):e5.

[33] Stephensen H, Andersson N, Eklund A, et al . Objective B wave analysis in 55 patients with non-communicating and communicat ing hydrocephalus. *J. Neurol. Neurosurg. Psychiatry.* 2005,76(7):965-70.

[34] Wraige E, Chandler C, Pohl KR. Idiopathic intracranial hypertension: is papilloedema inevitable? *Arch. Dis. Child.* 2002 ;87(3):223-4.

Chapter VIII

Intracranial Hypertension Classification

The most used classification of intracranial hypertension is the classification into:

- ICH generated by expansive intracranial lesions (tumors, hematomas, etc.), and
- ICH generated by a different illness than the intracranial space replacing process, also called pseudomotor cerebri.

The descriptive presentation of the intracranial hypertension differentiates two groups: the secondary intracranial hypertension, with an increase in the intracranial pressure generated by an obvious cause (tumor, cerebral venous thrombosis, meningitis, etc.) and the idiopathic intracranial hypertension without an identifiable cause. [1,2,3,5]

The descriptive classification of the clinical forms of intracranial hypertension includes:

1. Intracranial hypertension of a tumor cause, which depends on the tumor location and on the extension of the intracranial tumor.
2. Intracranial hypertension in expansive non-tumor intracranial lesions, which depends on the location of the lesion based on the circulation of the cerebrospinal fluid and on the impact on the venous circulation.
3. Intracranial hypertension in traumatic brain injury
4. Intracranial hypertension in congenital malformations, which lead to intracranial hypertension due to disorders of the cerebrospinal fluid.
5. Intracranial hypertension in hypertensive encephalopathy
6. Intracranial hypertension in the cerebral-vascular ischemic illness
7. Intracranial hypertension in cerebral venous thrombosis
8. Intracranial hypertension in obstructive internal hydrocephalus
9. Intracranial hypertension due to a decrease in the resorption of the cerebrospinal fluid
10. The intracranial hypertension generated by a diffuse cerebral suffering caused by endogenous or exogenous toxics, often with an acute beginning.
11. Idiopathic intracranial hypertension

Depending on the clinical stage and on the development, intracranial hypertension may occur as:

- an infraclinical stage – when the intracranial pressure is high, but below the normality threshold. If the intracranial pressure usually has values of up to 8-12 mm Hg, manifesting daily variations in the value range between 4-6 mmHg and 10-12 mm Hg, the occurrence of a pathologic cerebral process can cause the increase in the intracranial pressure of approximately 15 - 17 mmHg without establishing a clinical symptomatology due to the pressure increase.
- the clinical stage of an intracranial hypertension syndrome corresponds to intracranial pressure increases of up to 20 mm Hg, which is considered to be the normality threshold; this is the compensation period of intracranial pressure increases ~~on~~ for illnesses that evolve with an intracranial hypertension.
- the clinical illness stage or the intracranial hypertension as an illness, when the intracranial pressure increases exceed the normal threshold values, of approximately 20 mm Hg. At this stage the compensation mechanisms of these intracranial pressure increases have been exceeded.

The intracranial hypertension as an illness can include:

- an initial period when the intracranial pressure increases oscillate around the normal threshold value of 20 mm Hg, or the intracranial pressure increase is very slow. The compensation of the ICP increases is exceeded, but the situation is reversible under appropriate therapy. Cerebral circulatory disorders may occur. The clinical presentationof the intracranial hypertension syndrome is complete, and the symptoms are major ones.
- the state period, which corresponds to significant increases (sometimes sudden increases) in the intracranial pressure, with the occurrence of the cerebral hernia and of the brainstem ischemia, as well as with the clinical presentationof aggravation and coma. The etiological therapy, together with the decreasing therapy of increased intracranial pressure, also including the surgical decompression with disengagement if necessary, can sometimes lead to the amelioration of the clinical state.
- the final period – when the cerebral hernia or the massive ischemia of the cerebral parenchyma or of the brainstem have caused irreversible lesions.

The evolution of the ICH as an illness in its three stages is determined by

- the increasing speed of the intracranial pressure up to the normal threshold and then above the normal threshold,
- the maximum values of the intracranial pressure and the length of time for which the increased pressure values are maintained, and
- the frequency of the pathologic increases in intracranial pressure.

The classification of the intracranial hypertension is currently based on etiopathogenic and clinical criteria, and four forms have been identified:

- parenchymatous intracranial hypertension,
- vascular intracranial hypertension,
- intracranial hypertension due to disorders of the cerebrospinal fluid dynamics, and
- idiopathic intracranial hypertension.

1. Parenchymatous Intracranial Hypertension

It can occur in:

- expansive intracranial lesions: brain tumors, intracranial hematoma, brain abscesses, brain hydatid cyst etc.,
- posttraumatic brain edema,
- hypoxic brain edema by posttraumatic secondary cerebral ischemia or from sub-arachnoid hemorrhage,
- general intoxications with neurotoxins (endogenous or exogenous), etc.

The primary cerebral cause and the pathogenic mechanisms are known; usually, a supplementary intracranial volume occurs, then the brain edema, which develops in parallel to the ICP increase or the brain edema is secondary to a diffuse cerebral lesion. The intrinsic cerebral etiology and the primary endocranial modifications of volume (new expansive or compressive volume, hypoxic or traumatic brain edema) produce the initial parenchymatous lesion. The evolution of this lesion causes the intracranial pressure increase; subsequently, the clinical and paraclinical characteristic presentation of the syndrome and then of the decompensated ICH occur. The parenchymatous intracranial hypertension can have a complete evolution, to the acute form with a brainstem ischemia or a cerebral herniation. [1,3,5]

2. Vascular Intracranial Hypertension

The etiology is represented by disorders of the sanguine, cerebral or extra-cerebral circulation, which leads to the ICP increase. The volume of the cerebral parenchyma increases by means of the brain edema or by the increase in the brain blood volume (brain swelling), leading to the increase in the intracranial pressure. The increase in the cerebral sanguine volume is secondary to an increased intracranial arterial sanguine contribution, or it occurs because of the decrease or blockage of the venous drainage. In this case, a decrease in the resorption of the cerebrospinal fluid ~~is~~ also happens. [1,3,5,6]

Two types of changes happen at the level of the nervous parenchyma:

- brain edema due to water accumulation in the cerebral parenchyma, and
- brain swelling, with an increase in the volume of the cerebral parenchyma by vascular dilatation.

The vascular intracranial hypertension is produced by:

- the decreased venous drainage and the blocked resorption of the intracranial cerebrospinal fluid in the cerebral venous thrombosis, thrombosis of the superior sagittal sinus, cerebral thrombophlebites, mastoiditis ("otitic hydrocephalus" described by Symonds – thrombosis of venous sinuses, secondary to otomastoiditis), shunting of the superior longitudinal sinus in certain arterio-venous malformations, etc., or extra-cranial in illnesses that may lead to a cervical or thoracic venous blockage.
- an extremely rapid arterial sanguine contribution, which exceeds the capacity of the cerebral venous drainage, in the hypertensive encephalopathy with congestive brain edematization and with an extracellular hydrostatic brain edema (by ultra-filtration);
- in the decrease of the cerebral sanguine contribution by cerebral ischemia with secondary ischemic brain edema as in the ischemic stroke caused by the occlusion or the stenosis of the great cerebral vessels, with a severe form of massive ischemic stroke within the territory of the middle cerebral artery.

3. Intracranial Hypertension Due to Disorders in the Dynamics of the Cerebrospinal Fluid

The normal dynamics of the cerebrospinal fluid is represented by the circulation of the cerebrospinal fluid from the moment of formation at the level of the choroid plexuses and until the passage of the cerebrospinal fluid into the venous circulation.

The dynamic disorders of the cerebrospinal fluid can be:

- circulation disorders of the cerebrospinal fluid from formation till resorption, and
- passage disorders of the cerebrospinal fluid in the venous drainage system (resorption).

The circulation disorders of the cerebrospinal fluid occur if there is an obstacle at the level of the fluid route (ventricular system, magna cistern, and basal cisterns) due to the existence of a ventricular or paraventricular tumor, intra-ventricular hemorrhage or various obstructions of the Sylvian aqueduct. There is a dilatation of the ventricular system segments that are superjacent to the obstruction, while the clinical presentationand the evolution belong to the obstructive internal hydrocephalus.

The resorption disorders of the cerebrospinal fluid occur in acute meningitis, subarachnoid hemorrhage, meningeal carcinomatosis, chronic meningitis in sarcoidosis, etc.

A thickening of the leptomeninx occurs, leading to the blockage of the Pacchioni arachnoid corpuscles and the decreased absorption of the cerebrospinal fluid. The cerebrospinal fluid accumulates in the ventricular system generating a communicating hydrocephalus, with a periventricular, hydrocephalic brain edema and with an intracranial hypertension syndrome, usually a sub-acute one (called “meningeal intracranial hypertension”). The clinical presentation and the intracranial pressure increase are similar to the intracranial hypertension syndrome in cases of obstructed circulation of the cerebrospinal fluid. [1,3,5]

4. Idiopathic Intracranial Hypertension

It has also been called pseudotumor cerebri, essential or cryptogenic ICH because the etiology could not be identified. The idiopathic intracranial hypertension occurs in certain endocrine illnesses, various metabolic disorders or hematological diseases. The supposed physio-pathologic mechanisms have been thought to be disorders in the secretion and absorption of the cerebrospinal fluid, while the ICP increase is secondary to the decreased absorption of the cerebrospinal fluid, without the occurrence of hydrocephalus. The brain edema may be generated by the so-called non-specific “associated factors” that induce the ICP increase, but with no possibility of establishing an etiologic relation. The auto-regulation of the cerebral blood circulation compensates the ICP increase and it maintains the cerebral blood flux.

The most recent pathogenic hypothesis for the idiopathic intracranial hypertension is based on the dynamics of the intracranial fluid circuits that explain the maintenance of the auto-regulation of the cerebral circulation and of the cerebral blood flux. In the idiopathic ICH, certain indeterminate pathological conditions cause injuries of the brain-blood barrier, resulting in a hyper-production of interstitial fluid and the occurrence of the extracellular brain edema. The cerebrospinal fluid is normally secreted at the level of the choroid plexuses. The increased pressure of the cerebral parenchyma is equalized by the pressure of the cerebrospinal fluid due to increased exchanges of the interstitial fluid towards the cerebrospinal fluid at the trans-ependyma and pial trans-cerebral level. Afterwards, the increased resorption of the cerebrospinal fluid is produced, as well as a rapid venous return. Due to this circulation of the interstitial fluid and the increased resorption of the cerebrospinal fluid, the increased intracranial pressure does not affect the cerebral circulation, which is within normal limits. The trans-ependymal and trans-pial circuit of the interstitial fluid towards the cerebrospinal fluid is an efficient compensating mechanism in idiopathic intracranial hypertension, and it allows the cerebral circulatory auto-regulation.

The idiopathic intracranial hypertension occurs due to the impact on the brain-blood barrier of various indeterminate causes, with a hyper-production of interstitial fluid and a secondary extracellular brain edema, with increased exchanges from the interstitial fluid towards the cerebrospinal fluid at the trans-ependymal and pial trans-cerebral level; subsequently, there is an increased resorption of the cerebrospinal fluid, and a rapid venous efflux (Iencean, 2003 , 2004). The idiopathic ICH evolves into an incomplete ICH syndrome, despite the increased ICP values and the presence of the papillary edema. [1,2,3,3,5]

The intracranial hypertension syndrome can also occur as a form of transition among these four forms of ICH when several pathogenic mechanisms coexist, acting simultaneously or successively; for example, the ICH syndrome can be induced by several concomitant pathogenic mechanisms of the brain edema in: bacillary meningo-encephalitis, neoplasia, hydro-electrolytic disorders, diabetic ceto-acidosis, the dialysis disequilibrium syndrome, post-resuscitation cerebral syndrome, fulminating hepatic failure, etc.

References

[1] Iencean St M A new classification and a synergetical pattern in intracranial hypertension . Medical Hypotheses , 2002 Feb;58(2):159-63.

[2] Iencean St M Idiopathic intracranial hypertension and idiopathic normal pressure hydrocephalus: diseases with opposite pathogenesis? Medical Hypotheses. 2003 ;61(5-6):526-8.

[3] Iencean St M Pattern of increased intracranial pressure and classification of intracranial hypertension. Journal of Medical Sciences, 2004, vol.4,Nr.1 :52- 58

[4] Iencean St M Simultaneous hypersecretion of CSF and of brain interstitial fluid causes idiopathic intracranial hypertension. Medical Hypotheses. 2003 ;61(5-6):529-32.

[5] Iencean St M Classification and essential conditions of decompensation in intracranial hypertension Rom J Neurosurgery 2004,Vol. I No. 1 January–June, pp. 3-13

[6] Iencean St M Vascular intracranial hypertension, J Med Sciences 2004, 4, 4 : 276 – 281

Chapter IX

Differential Diagnosis

1.Clinical Differential Diagnosis

The clinical differential diagnosis of the intracranial hypertension depends on the clinical state, especially in the case of:

- a conscious patient, with symptoms that announce a cerebral condition, or
- a patient with conscience disorders or who is in a coma.

If the patient is conscious and presents a symptomatology that is characteristic for a cerebral suffering, the differential diagnosis is the one of the isolated ICH signs, but which may occur in other illnesses too:

- cephalea,
- papillary edema,
- vomiting,
- psychic disorders.

The association between cephalea and the eye fundus modifications is significant for the intracranial hypertension. The psychic disorders and/or the vomiting complete the clinical presentation, which becomes pathognomic for intracranial hypertension. [3,5]

A clinical presentation that is very similar to the one of intracranial hypertension is present in the intracranial hypotension syndrome. The postural cephalea is accompanied by vomiting, followed by neurological disorders, usually minor ones. The symptomatology can escalate and psychic disorders may occur. The outlining of cranial-cerebral, spinal or neurosurgical exploration traumatic antecedents (lumbar puncture, surgery) facilitates the diagnosis. There is also a form of spontaneous or idiopathic intracranial hypotension, whose etiology remains unrevealed yet.

The intracranial hypotension lacks the papillary edema and the diagnosis can be established by means of magnetic resonance. [3,4,5]

Sometimes, there is only one isolated symptom, which imposes a clinical differential diagnosis, based on a thorough anamnesis, correlated to the performance of a neurological examination that may guide subsequent explorations. The apparently isolated symptom is often a dominating symptom, and the clinical examination establishes the presence of the quasi-complete clinical syndrome, with the other signs present, but of a reduced intensity, and to which the patient or their family grants no significance whatsoever.

The concretization of the differential diagnosis of cephalea underlines first of all the starting characteristics:

- acute cephalea, which may be localized or generalized,
- chronic, progressive or constant cephalea,
- recurrent cephalea, with periodic worsening or random paroxysm.

The cephalea must be differentiated from facial pains, and the clinical examination shows whether the cephalea is localized or generalized.

In intracranial hypertension with a progressive development, cephalea is diffuse, permanent, with periodic exacerbations and with slow or rapid worsening. It is more intense in the morning, in parallel to the nocturnal increase in the intracranial pressure, and it partially or sufficiently diminishes after a vomiting episode. Usual analgesics have a limited effect. Depending on how rapid the evolution of the causal disorder is, and on how the intracranial hypertension is installed, cephalea generally has a progressive character, with permanent worsening of the intensity and the increase in the frequency of the hyperalgic episodes.

In contrast to this evolutionary character of cephalea in intracranial hypertension, cephalea in other medical conditions maintains its characteristics for long periods. [3,5,7,9]

The differential diagnosis is based on:

- migraine cephalea: classic migraine, ophthalmologic migraine, etc.,
- cephalea by meningeal inflammatory processes: meningitis, sub-arachnoid hemorrhage of various etiologies, etc.,
- cephalea present in cervical vertebral rheumatologic disorders,
- cephalea as an accompanying symptom in various internal illnesses, etc.
- facial pains with frontal-temporal irradiation, of ocular, sinus, dental, otic etiologies, etc.,
- cranial-facial neuralgias, etc.

The papillary edema requires the differentiation from other ophthalmologic disorders by the ophthalmologist: inflammatory papillitis, hypermetropic pseudo-nephritis, etc.

Although included in the classic pathognomic triad for the intracranial hypertension syndrome, vomiting can occur at a later stage in the evolution of the intracranial hypertension, and its frequency depends on the patient's age and on the cause of the ICP increase.

The differentiation from a digestive disorder accompanied by vomiting is provided by a thorough anamnesis and paraclinical exploration.

Psychic disorders are frequent in the intracranial hypertension syndrome, and there can be problems related to the differential diagnosis. The anamnesis identifies the existence of certain symptoms of an organic illness, and the neurological examination shows discrete signs that require cerebral explorations. In the context of certain psychic disorders of different aspects and intensity in the clinical presentationof the cranial-cerebral organic lesions, many psychic illnesses need an exclusion diagnosis, based on a cerebral computer tomography or a cerebral magnetic resonance exploration.

In the case of a patient in a coma, whose anamnesis data and clinical examination raise the suspicion of an endocranial etiopathogeny, the paraclinical exploration is immediately performed by a cerebral computer tomography, perhaps by a cerebral MNR, underlining the diagnosis.

2.Diagnosis of Forms of Intracranial Hypertension

The four forms of intracranial hypertension differ from one another in etiology, pathogenic mechanisms including the formation of the brain edema, the type of intracranial pressure increase and the effect on the cerebral circulation and the evolution method. [1,2,3,5]

The parenchymatous intracranial hypertension has the following specific characteristics:

- Known etiology: it occurs in the expansive intracranial processes (cerebral tumors, intracranial hematoma, cerebral abscesses, etc.), in the traumatic brain edema, in cerebral ischemia with hypoxic brain edema, in general intoxications with neurotoxins (endogenous or exogenous), etc.,
- The brain edema (cytotoxic, vasogenic or mix) may be a perifocal edema,
- The intracranial pressure increases rapidly and it exceeds the normal threshold value of 20 mm Hg. The increased intracranial pressure reduces the cerebral circulation auto-regulation and there are pressure differences between the cerebrospinal compartments. The increased ICP has a short period of action until decompensation.
- The paraclinical explorations, by CT or cerebral MRI reveal the endocranial lesion.
- Complete development towards decompensated ICH by cerebral hernia or by brainstem ischemia.

The intracranial hypertension can occur in cerebral-vascular illnesses due to blood cerebral or extra-cerebral circulatory disorders, which modify the dynamics of intracranial fluids and lead to the increase in the intracranial pressure. [3,5]

- The etiology refers to a cerebral or general vascular illness,
- The brain edema is present (vasogenic edema), whether in one sector or generalized,
- A moderate increase in the intracranial pressure occurs, exceeding the critical value of 20 mm Hg; usually there are no ICP differences between the cerebrospinal compartments,

- The auto-regulation of the cerebral circulation is influenced first of all by the vascular illness, and then there is the action of the increased intracranial pressure,
- Generally, there is a long period of action performed by the increased intracranial pressure until decompensation occurs; the exception is represented by the malignant middle cerebral artery infarction with rapid evolution towards decompensation,
- The paraclinical explorations establish the absence of an expansive intracranial process and they reveal the vascular disorder (venous sinus thrombosis, hypertensive encephalopathy or the cerebral ischemic infarct),
- Usually the evolution is towards an ICH syndrome, without decompensation, and with the same exception of the complete ischemic infarct of middle cerebral artery,

The intracranial hypertension due to disorders of the cerebrospinal fluid dynamics represents the intracranial pressure increase caused by the disorders of the cerebrospinal fluid circulation from formation and till its passage into the venous circulation.

In case of circulation disorders of the cerebrospinal fluid from formation to the resorption place:

- The etiology is known and it consists of an obstruction of the cerebrospinal fluid circulation,
- An obstructive hydrocephalus occurs quite rapidly with a periventricular edema or with a generalized brain edema,
- The increase in the intracranial pressure is rapid, exceeding the normal threshold value of 20 mm Hg; the increased ICP reduces the auto-regulation of the cerebral circulation. There are ICP differences between the cerebrospinal compartments. The increased intracranial pressure has a limited period of action because the decompensation can occur within a short period of time.
- Paraclinical explorations establish the presence of an obstacle throughout the circulation of the cerebrospinal fluid till resorption (ventricular or paraventricular tumor, intra-ventricular hemorrhage, etc),
- The evolution is complete towards the form of decompensated intracranial hypertension,

In case of resorption disorders of the cerebrospinal fluid (venous drainage):

- The etiology is known: acute meningitis, in subarachnoid hemorrhage of traumatic brain injury, in intracranial aneurysms, etc, in meningeal carcinomatosis, in chronic meningitis of sarcoidosis, etc.,
- A communicating hydrocephalus is produced with periventricular hydrocephalic edema or with a generalized brain edema,
- There is a moderate increase in the intracranial pressure, exceeding the normal threshold value of 20 mm Hg; there are no ICP differences between cerebrospinal compartments. The action period of the increased intracranial pressure is variable and it depends on the maximum ICP values, which may be compensated,

- There is an inflammatory vasculitis that can have impacts on the auto-regulation of the cerebral circulation,
- Paraclinical explorations exclude other types of intracranial hypertension and they reveal the inflammatory meningeal context (infectious, mechanical, etc.),
- The evolution depends on etiology and it usually heads towards a complete or incomplete ICH syndrome

The idiopathic intracranial hypertension consists of the intracranial pressure increase in the absence of an expansive intracranial process, of hydrocephalus, of an intracranial infection, of dural venous thrombosis or of hypertensive encephalopathy. Therefore, the idiopathic ICH is an exclusion diagnosis in a specific etiologic and clinical context.

- The etiology is not specified or the involvement of various unspecific factors is not accepted, factors that have been named “associated factors”,
- There is an extracellular brain edema, which is balanced by the intra-ventricular pressure,
- The intracranial pressure increases very slowly, exceeding the normal threshold value and reaching very high values of up to 60-80 mm Hg, and it maintains these high values for long periods of time. ICP is constantly increased in all the cerebrospinal compartments.
- Despite the very high increase in the intracranial pressure, the auto-regulation of the cerebral circulation is maintained by the intense absorption mechanism of the cerebrospinal fluid and of the parenchymatous interstitial fluid.
- Paraclinical explorations exclude any expansive intracranial process, as well as any other form of intracranial hypertension; the thrombosis of the endocranial venous sinuses are included in the vascular ICH,
- The evolution goes towards an incomplete ICH syndrome. There is a disparity between the minimum clinical presentationcompared to the very high values of the intracranial pressure and the presence of the papillary edema. There may be a decrease in the visual acuity, which has led to the renunciation of the old term of “benign” intracranial hypertension

3. Diagnosis of the ICH Clinical Stage

The evolution of the intracranial hypertension includes three stages, which are characterized by:

- defined values of the intracranial pressure at the moment it passes to the next stage, and
- specific clinical symptoms generated by modifications of the volume-pressure relation.

These stages may be consecutive from developmental point of view, or the development can stop at one of them, depending on the etiopathogeny of the illness or on the efficiency of the applied therapy:

a. the ICP increase above the normal values of up to 15-16 mm Hg is an alarm sign, but the clinical symptomatology is non-characteristic, with the existence of several minor psychic signs: asthenia, perhaps depression, apathy etc.
b. the ICP increase progressively exceeds the critical value of 20 mm Hg, with the occurrence of the ICH syndrome; the ICH syndrome evolves depending on the etiology and on maintaining the auto-regulation of the cerebral sanguine circulation. The compensating mechanisms may block the pressure-time fluctuation for a while, so that the clinical presentationincludes the progressive start of the symptomatology. The pathogenic mechanisms that lead to intracranial pressure increases in the idiopathic intracranial hypertension allow the maintenance of the cerebral circulation auto-regulation, and therefore, the decompensation of this ICH form is not achieved.
c. the compensating mechanisms are exceeded, and they may no longer block the development towards the acute stage; therefore, the acute critical ICP values eventually cause the alteration of the circulatory auto-regulation.

The acute stage of the intracranial hypertension has a characteristic clinical chart, and the diagnosis and therapy must be fast in order to hinder the clinical decompensation.

The first and the second stages are reversible, while the third stage corresponds to a phase of maximum instability, when the decompensation with clinical aggravation is caused by a brainstem ischemia or by brain herniation, which causes irreversible cerebral lesions.[2,3,4,6,8,9]

References

[1] Distelmaiera F, Senglerb U, Messing-Juengerc M et al. Pseudotumor cerebri as an important differential diagnosis of papilledema in children,Brain and Development ,28, 3, 2006, 190-195
[2] Friedman, DI. Papilledema and pseudotumor cerebri. Ophthal Clin North Am 2001; 14:129.
[3] Iencean St M A new classification and a synergetical pattern in intracranial hypertension Medical Hypotheses , 2002 Feb;58(2):159-63.
[4] Iencean St M Idiopathic intracranial hypertension and idiopathic normal pressure hydrocephalus: diseases with opposite pathogenesis? Medical Hypotheses. 2003 ;61(5-6):526-8.
[5] Iencean St M Pattern of increased intracranial pressure and classification of intracranial hypertension. Journal of Medical Sciences, 2004, vol.4,Nr.1 :52- 58
[6] Iencean St M Simultaneous hypersecretion of CSF and of brain interstitial fluid causes idiopathic intracranial hypertension. Medical Hypotheses. 2003 ;61(5-6):529-32.

[7] Iencean St M Classification and essential conditions of decompensation in intracranial hypertension Rom J Neurosurgery 2004,Vol. I No. 1 January–June, pp. 3-13

[8] Iencean St M Vascular intracranial hypertension, J Med Sciences 2004, 4, 4 : 276 – 281

[9] Sylaja PN, Ahsan Moosa NV, Radhakrishnan K et al Differential diagnosis of patients with intracranial sinus venous thrombosis related isolated intracranial hypertension from those with idiopathic intracranial hypertension. J Neurol Sci. 2003 , 15;215(1-2):9-12.

Chapter X

Parenchymatous Intracranial Hypertension

General Data

The parenchymatous intracranial hypertension is the intracranial pressure increase caused by the intracranial volume modifications due to an intrinsic parenchymatous lesion (expansive intra-parenchymatous lesion, brain edema, etc.) or an extrinsic lesion (tumor, traumatic, infectious extra-parenchymatous compression, etc.). The primary cerebral lesion and the secondary endocranial volume changes (expansive or compressive new volume, hypoxic or traumatic brain edema, etc.) cause disorders of the intracranial pressure equilibrium mechanisms. The infraclinical stage includes the compensating mechanisms of the intracranial pressure increase and, if these mechanisms are exceeded by the pressure increase, the characteristic clinical and paraclinical charts of the intracranial hypertension syndrome are shown. [6,20,21]

The parenchymatous intracranial hypertension develops depending on the existing etiology, on how rapidly the parenchymatous lesion extends, on the compensating mechanisms of the pressure increases, and on the efficiency of the medical and/or neurosurgical treatment.

The development of the parenchymatous intracranial hypertension includes:

- an incipient ICH syndrome,
- a compensated ICH syndrome, or
- a complete development till decompensation – the acute form with brainstem ischemia or with cerebral hernia.

The parenchymatous intracranial hypertension can occur in:

- the intracranial space-replacing lesions: cerebra tumors, hematomas, cerebral tumors, intracranial hematomas, cerebral abscesses, intracranial cystic lesions, etc.,
- the traumatic brain edema,

- the hypoxic brain edema through posttraumatic secondary cerebral ischemia or in sub-arachnoid hemorrhage,
- general intoxications with neurotoxins: endogenous or exogenous.

The parenchymatous intracranial hypertension varies in its starting manner, intensity of symptoms and development, which depend on:

- the nature of the lesion, which determines the development speed and the effect of the lesion on the neighbouring cerebral parenchyma (brain edema),
- the location of the lesion, which can involve the sector or integral cerebral parenchyma (encephalitis, generalized brain edema), depending on the involvement of the cerebral vessels or of the anatomic paths of circulation of the cerebrospinal fluid. The vascular compression causes ischemic disorders and the blockage of the cerebrospinal fluid circulation can lead to an obstructive hydrocephalus.

Depending on these characteristics, intracranial disorders may present a specific, focal symptomatology, (epileptic crises, motor and sensorial deficits, etc.) or general symptoms (asthenia, cephalea, psychic disorders, endocrine disorders, etc.) or they may start as an intracranial hypertension syndrome. There are significant differences from the point of view of evolution, prognosis and therapy between intracranial disorders that start as an intracranial hypertension syndrome and those starting as a focal or non-characteristic symptomatology, and which subsequently present an ICH syndrome. [20,21,22]

A distinction is made between:

- the parenchymatous intracranial hypertension with an acute start, and
- the parenchymatous intracranial hypertension with an progressive start.

I. Acute Parenchymatous Intracranial Hypertension

The parenchymatous intracranial hypertension with an acute start occurs when the intracranial pressure increase is very fast due to the precipitated lesion production, or to the sudden surpassing of the pressure compensating mechanisms in the case of an intracranial lesion with a progressive infraclinical evolution. The acute ICH due to a severe cranial-cerebral lesion is typical for severe traumatic brain injury, but it may also occur in another acutely installed cerebral suffering, such as the intra-parenchymatous hematomas formed on the high blood pressurebackground or the breaking of a cerebral vascular malformation, etc. In these disorders, the starting symptoms are represented by the symptoms of the decompensated intracranial hypertension. [21,22]

A. Acute Intracranial Hypertension in Traumatic Brain Injury

The traumatic brain injury are produced via the action of a traumatic force on the cephalic extremity. The action of the traumatic agent is direct or the traumatic force can be transmitted by means of other anatomic structures (the backbone) up to the level of the head. After the impact, the cerebral traumatic effects occur by means of a contact mechanism or through inertial mechanisms (mechanisms of the acceleration / deceleration type).

Classification of Traumatic Brain Injury

The classification of the traumatic brain injury presented below is an integrating classification, according to its authors' acknowledged intention; it is conceived before the generalization of the efficient explorations from the end of the twentieth century, and it attempts to achieve a correlation between the clinical aspect with a pathologic anatomy and the evolution. [5,20]

According to this classification, traumatic brain injury produce:

A. Immediate traumatic effects:

I. Primary: their occurrence is compulsory and immediately after the impact; they are specifically traumatic:

a. The cerebral commotion is the primary traumatic effect manifested by a short and sudden loss of the state of consciousness,which is completely reversible, it is a diffuse brain injury.
b. The cerebral contusion is the primary traumatic effect induced by direct vascular perturbations, or vasomotor reflexes with various degrees of hemorrhage in the cerebral parenchyma, generating hypoxia and hemorrhagic lesions; it is a focal cerebral lesion.
c. The cerebral lacerations is a focal primary traumatic effect, a lesion with a destructive character, and it consists of the lack of continuity of the brain parenchyma surface. It may be: direct brain lacerations – by a foreign body or a cranial-cerebral wound – by a splinter of bone from the internal plate indirect brain laceration – by the cortical injury against the endocranial bone relief.

Open traumatic brain injury with great septic potential: - cranial-cerebral wounds (direct cerebral dilaceration) - fistulas of cerebrospinal fluid

II. Secondary: they do not necessarily happen, and they are not constantly specific traumatic

a. The traumatic hematomas are well-limited intracranial blood collections, with a compressive effect on the cerebral parenchyma:

- extra-cerebral - extradural hematoma
- subdural hematoma
- intradural hematoma
- intra-cerebral - intra-parenchymatous hematoma
- intra-ventricular hematoma

b. The intracranial fluid collections – are compressive focal lesions:
- dura mater hygroma

III. General or subsequent: these are not specifically traumatic, they are diffuse lesions:

a. Brain edema,
b. Cerebro-ventricular collapse

IV. Septic complications of open traumatic brain injury

a. localized lesions: cerebral abscesses, cerebral fungus
b. diffuse lesions – meningoencephalitis,

B. Delayed posttraumatic effects:

- Evolutionary – Posttraumatic encephalopathy
  – Posttraumatic epilepsy
  – Progressive hydrocephalus
- Traumatic sequels: aphasia, hemiplegia, epilepsy, etc.

In 1982, Gennarelli classifies cerebral lesions into focal lesions with surgical indication and diffuse cerebral lesions that do not have surgical indications, no matter how serious they are.

In 1991, Marshall and his collaborators define cerebral lesions based on the cranial-cerebral computer tomography exploration and based on:

- the aspect of the perimesencephalic cisterns: compressed, absent;
- the movement of the median line structures (measured in mm);
- the presence of the intra-parenchymatous hemorrhages and the measurement of their volume;
- the presence or the absence of the expansive processes with surgical indication.

The classification of traumatisms based on these criteria is as follows:

I. Diffuse traumatic lesions

Type I (degree I) – without pathologic computer tomography modifications

Type II (degree II) – perimesencephalic cisterns are present, there may be a movement of the median line ≤ 5 mm, there may hyper-dense lesions with volume < 25 cm^3

Type III (degree III) – brain edema present with the compression or absence of perimesencephalic cisterns, the movement of the median line is ≤ 5 mm , there may be hyper-dense lesions with volume < 25 cm^3

Type IV (degree IV) – diffuse lesions occur, the movement of the median line is > 5 mm there are hyperdense lesions with volume < 25 cm^3

II. Focal lesions include – contusive-hemorrhagic focuses,
- brain laceration
- axial and extra-axial hematomas,
- localized sub-arachnoid hemorrhage,
- direct injury of cranial nerves.

Depending on how intense and serious the lesions are, and on the clinical presentation assessed on the Glasgow scale (Glasgow Coma Scale), in 1986 Miller proposed the following classification:

1. Minor traumatic brain injury, which correspond to a GCS score = 15-13. They are differentiated, according to how serious they are, into:

- degree 0 – without loss of consciousness, with local pains, ecchymoses,
- degree 0 with risk – in case of alcoholism, in old people, patients with epileptic antecedents,
- degree 1 – minimum loss of consciousness, with amnesia, cephalea,
- degree 2 - GCS score 14-13 and loss of consciousness

2. Moderate traumatic brain injury correspond to a GCS score = 12- 9, patients have had a loss of consciousness of more than 5-10 min; clinically, they present a confusion syndrome, somnolence, the focal syndrome

3. Severe traumatic brain injury correspond to a GCS score ≤ 8 and patients are in coma:

- GCS = 8 1st degree coma
- GCS = 7-6 2nd degree coma
- GCS = 5-4 3rd degree coma
- GCS = 3 4th degree coma

Pathogenesis of Intracranial Hypertension in Traumatic Brain Injury

The pathogenesis of traumatic brain injury includes the action of the traumatic factor and the transmission of the lesional force to the cephalic extremity, as well as the reaction of the endocranial structures to the action of the traumatic agent. [20,21,22]

The occurrence of the intracranial hypertension syndrome and the clinical deterioration are caused by the way endocranial lesions are produced and by the rapidity with which the endocranial volume is exceeded beyond the limit that provides the pressure compensation.

Immediately after the action of the aggressive agent, the cerebral response is the primary traumatic lesion. The latter is the result of the tissue deformation induced by the mechanical forces at the moment of the traumatism, producing lesions of the blood vessels, of neurons and their axons and of the glial cells. Lesions may be unique, multiple or diffuse, and every type of lesion evolves differently depending on the injured structure and on the intensity of the lesion.

Depending on the interested component, the following reactions can occur:

- functional reaction, in cerebral commotion,
- neuronal and glial lesional reaction, causing a neuronal and a glial destruction,
- vascular lesional reaction:
    - vascular dilaceration, causing hemorrhages and hematomas,
    - thrombosis of the cerebral vessels with cerebral ischemia.

The immediate focal traumatic lesions are:

- vascular lesions that cause:
    - an intra-cerebral hemorrhage and intra-cerebral traumatic hematomas
    - subarachnoid traumatic hemorrhage
    - extradural, subdural traumatic hematomas
    - intra-ventricular hemorrhage
- brain contusion,
- brain laceration

and diffuse traumatic lesions:

- cerebral commotion, interpreted as a minimum form of diffuse axonal lesion,
- diffuse axonal lesion.
- diffuse vascular lesions

The posttraumatic diffuse vascular lesions are represented by multiple hemorrhagic focuses at the level of both cerebral hemispheres, especially in the white matter and at the level of the brainstem; they occur especially in severe cerebral traumatisms.

This type of lesion has mixed features since it combines the characteristics of the contusive focal lesion, but it occurs in extended areas of the cerebral parenchyma, which also grants it the features of diffuse traumatic lesion. [6,10,20]

The secondary traumatic cerebral lesions are the consequence of the physio-pathologic processes that commence at the moment of the traumatism, or which are produced by the primary traumatic lesion. At the cellular level, there is a hyper-metabolic response, the ATP concentration is reduced, free radicals occur and the peroxidases are activated; the dysfunction of the Ca^{2+} transport and of the Na^{+}-K^{+} pump happens with the occurrence of the capillary endothelial lesions and of the neuronal and glial cellular lesions.

There is a manifestation of:

- brain edema
- hypoxia, anoxia,
- brain swelling by paralytic vasodilatation,
- infectious complications,
- intracranial hematomas ,
- ventricular collapse, etc.

The occurrence of the cellular brain edema leads to the intracranial pressure increase; afterwards, there is a decrease in the cerebral perfusion pressure with the occurrence of the cerebral ischemia and of the extracellular oncotic brain edema, leading to a mixed brain edema. The intracranial pressure increase, non-compensated or non-treated, causes the installation of the intracranial hypertension syndrome.

Primary or secondary traumatic lesions cause the intracranial pressure increase through the increase in the endocranial volume due to:

1. - a supplementary volume added by:
- traumatic intra-parenchymatous hematoma
- extra-parenchymatous hematoma – subdural or extradural

2. - increase in the volume of the brain parenchyma due to:
- brain edema,
- brain swelling

The traumatic brain edema is a mixed brain edema and it occurs related to a focal lesion, a contusion or a brain laceration, as an initial perilesional brain edema, and which subsequently extends, and may eventually be generalized. Moreover, the brain edema may accompany a diffuse traumatic lesion, especially the posttraumatic diffuse vascular lesions, as an extracellular oncotic (vasogenic) brain edema. In the case of the diffuse axonal lesion, the occurrence of secondary axon lesions (secondary axotomy) is accompanied by an axonal edema at the level of the white cerebral matter and in the brainstem.

The brain swelling is caused by the disorder in the auto-regulation of the immediately posttraumatic cerebral circulation, manifested by paralytic vasodilatation and the occurrence of an extracellular brain edema of a hydrostatic type, by ultra-filtration (closed brain-blood barrier). If these disorders are not corrected, the extracellular oncotic (vasogenic) brain edema can also occur afterwards due to the severe alteration of the brain blood barrier (open brain-blood barrier).

The occurrence of the cerebral ischemic metabolic disorders represents one of the most important secondary posttraumatic effects. The direct traumatic cerebral vascular lesions, the vascular spasm caused by the sub-arachnoid traumatic hemorrhage, the traumatic brain edema and the traumatic congestive brain edematization cause the alteration of the mechanisms of cerebral circulatory auto-regulation, with the cerebral perfusion decrease and the occurrence of cerebral ischemia. There is an increased permeability of the cerebral capillaries (open brain-blood barrier) and the extracellular oncotic (vasogenic) brain edema is formed.The evolution is usually rapid with the extension of the brain edema and the ICP increase.

3. *- the increase in the volume of the CSF (acute posttraumatic hydrocephalus) through:*

- blocking the circulation of the cerebrospinal fluid by:
    - intra-ventricular haemorrhage,
    - hematoma in the posterior fosse,
    - cerebellum contusion with edema, blocking the 4th ventricle.
- blocking the resorption of the CSF in the sub-arachnoid hemorrhage.

The mechanisms, by means of which the acute posttraumatic hydrocephalus occurs, include it in the pathogenic form of intracranial hypertension caused by dynamic disorders of the cerebrospinal fluid.

The occurrence of the immediate posttraumatic acute intracranial hypertension depends on the speed of the increase in the supplementary endocranial volume or of the expansion of the cerebral parenchyma volume, and, therefore, on the speed of the intracranial pressure increase up to the normal threshold value of 20 mm Hg and then above this value. The ICH syndrome, which occurs and is decompensated in secondary traumatic lesions, is also dependent on the volume – intracranial pressure relation and on exceeding the compensating capacity of the intracranial pressure increase.

Clinical Presentation

The acute intracranial hypertension syndrome is caused by the parenchymatous lesions due to cerebral herniation and to ischemic lesions due to the surpassing of the compensation capacities of the endocranial volume increases. The acute intracranial hypertension manifests itself clinically either through diencephalic-mesencephalic suffering and then the suffering of the rest of the brainstem, which escalate gradually and speedily, or through the occurrence or aggravation of the focal syndrome. [4,5,10,16]

The clinical presentation includes:

- the preexisting symptoms that escalate a lot rapidly: cephalea, vomiting, psychic disorders, etc.;
- initial convulsive crises happen or their frequency and duration increases;
- the worsening or the occurrence of the pyramidal syndrome, the interest of the cranial nerves;
- consciousness disorders (somnolence) and coma.

Cushing describes the clinical presentationof the intracranial hypertension syndrome aggravation, which includes bradycardia, increase in the systemic blood pressure, and the occurrence of respiratory disorders.

The occurrence of the unilateral mydriasis represents an alarm signal in the clinical presentationof a supra-tentorial expansive lesion.

The presence of the syndrome of acute traumatic intracranial hypertension, which is clinically manifested through consciousness disorders and ~~a~~ through coma, indicate a severe cerebral suffering, and it represents a serious prognosis factor.

The coma may occur immediately at the moment of traumatism when the primary lesion:

- is extensive, it has a very rapid evolution and there is an exponential increase in the intracranial pressure,
- there is a hemorrhagic or ischemic lesion at the level of the brainstem, without the intracranial hypertension syndrome, or
- it is a diffuse lesion: a severe diffuse axonal lesion, which interest the mesencephalon, and which causes a coma without the ICH syndrome

The syndrome of acute intracranial hypertension, with a state of coma, may occur later, after the traumatic brain injury, in one of the following situations:

- there is the so-called “free interval”, which represents the period of time when the supplementary endocranial volume develops, establishing the non-compensated pressure increase, the secondary diffuse traumatic cerebral lesions (edema, ischemia, etc.) lead to the decompensation of the intracranial hypertension

- the secondary traumatic cerebral lesions (edema, hemorrhage, ischemia) generate lesions in the mesencephalon and a state of coma, without the intracranial hypertension syndrome.

The assessment of the consciousness-conscience disorders, as well as the motor and pupil examination has allowed the clinical classification of traumatic brain injury according to the intensity of seriousness of lesions. This evaluation is based on certain scales that allow a simple and precise testing: the Glagow scale (Glasgow Coma Scale) introduced by Teasdale and Jennett in 1974. The complementation of the Glasgow scale by the examination of the brainstem reflexes represents the Glasgow – Liège scale, which allows a more precise assessment of the neurological presentation and a prognosis evaluation.

The evolution and the prognosis of the acute traumatic intracranial hypertension depends on the way the syndrome had begun– immediately at the moment of traumatism or, if it is gradual, after the traumatism, depending on the period of time when the decompensation happens; on the maximum value reached by the pathological intracranial pressure and on the duration of the increased pressure values. The efficiency of the therapy is validated by the clinical amelioration depending on the recovering period to normal pressure values and on the possibility of recurring pressure increases to pathological values.

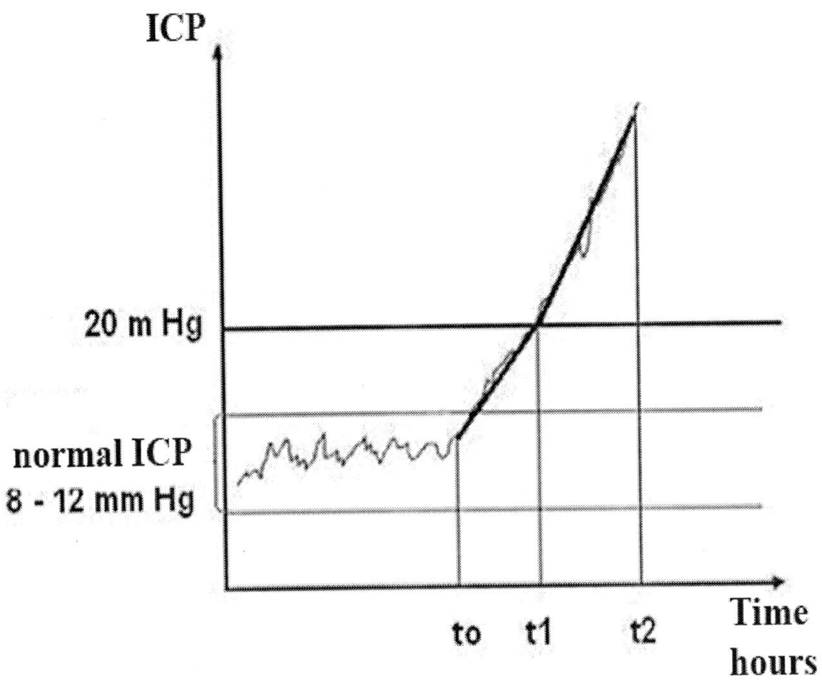

Figure 20(Repeated). The supra-acute increase in the intracranial pressure: the intervals to-t1 and t1-t2 are very short; the acute ICH due to the ICP increase practically happens at the moment of the traumatism

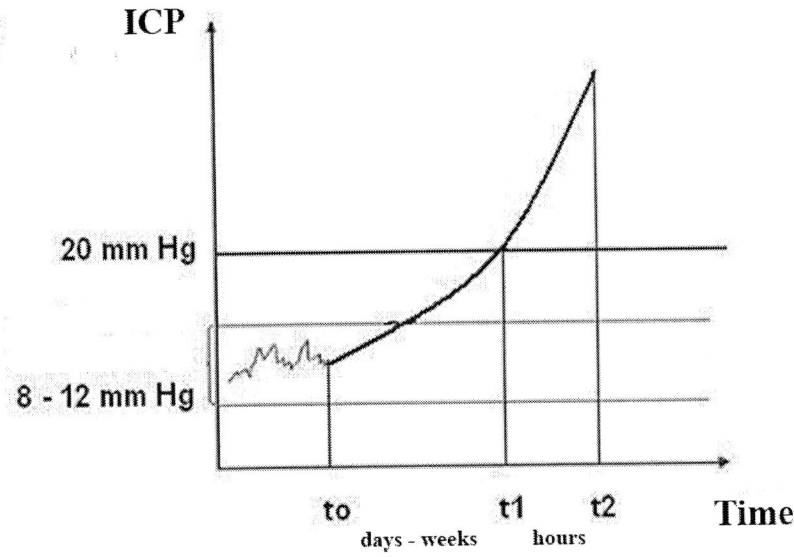

Figure 37. The acute increase in the intracranial pressure in the case of decompensated secondary traumatic cerebral lesions; the interval to-t1 is variable, but the interval 1-t2 is very short. The interval to-t1 is often presented as a "free interval" (the absence of an obvious symptomatology).

Paraclinical Explorations

In case of a patient with the suspicion of diagnosis of intracranial hypertension syndrome of traumatic cause, the recommended paraclinical investigation is the cerebral computer tomography. In case of severe traumatic brain injury, the computer tomography explorations must also include the cervical spine . MRI exploration reveals the non-hemorrhagic cerebral lesions better than the computer tomography, but it is not usually recommended in severe acute traumatic brain injury. The radiographic exploration of the cervical spine must be performed in all patients in traumatic coma; usually, the performance of cranial radiographies is not necessary after the cranial-cerebral computer tomography exploration. [21]

CT Scan

The CT scan is a rapid and non-invasive exploration, and it is performed without a contrast substance in traumatic brain injury. The cranial-cerebral computer tomography exploration is recommended in all severe traumatic brain injury, and it allows the observation of the neurosurgical lesions and of diffuse, hemorrhagic or edematous lesions. The normal cranial-cerebral computer tomography does not reveal any lesion: the absence of cranial fractures, the absence of a brain edema, the absence of the median line movement and the absence of hemorrhagic lesions. Sometimes, the cranial CT does not reveal small linear cranial fractures; moreover, a normal computer tomography image does not include a diffuse axonal lesion and it does not eliminate the possibility of a secondary hemorrhagic lesion. [6,10,17,23]

The pathological cranial-cerebral computer tomography images consist of:

- focal hemorrhagic lesions (cerebral contusion, brain laceration) or multiple hemorrhagic focuses,
- sub-arachnoid hemorrhage, intra-ventricular hemorrhage,
- unilateral or generalized brain edema, median line movement, compression on the ventricular system, compression or absence of the basal cisterns,
- acute subdural or extradural hematoma,
- traumatic intra-parenchymatous hematoma

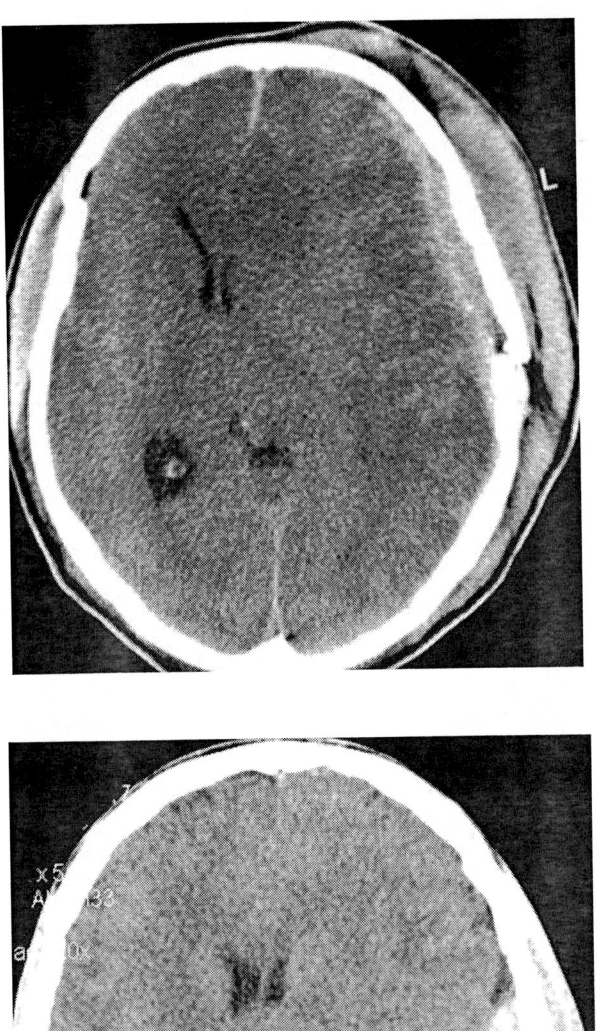

Figure 38. Bilateral cranial fracture with extradural Figure 39. Typical extradural hematoma, movement of hematoma under the left parietal fracture trajectory, ventricular system, acute traumatic, 2nd degree coma, with significant traumatic edema and with an acute Glasgow score 7. Traumatic ICH syndrome; 3rd degree coma, Glasgow score 5.

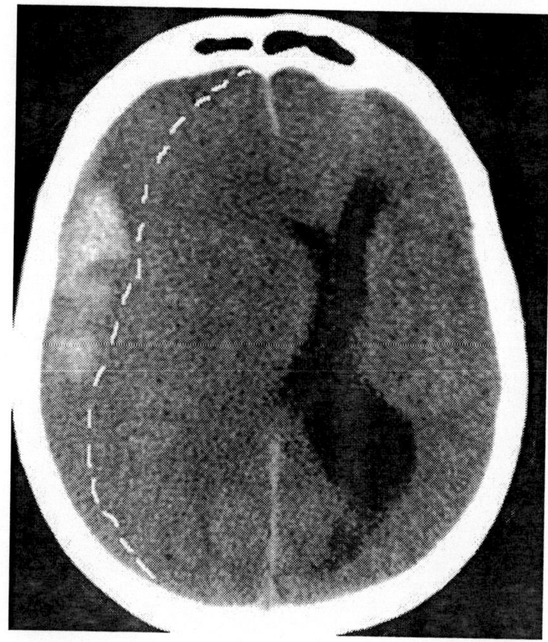

Figure 40. Right hemispheric subdural hematoma – the native cerebral CT image shows the very large movement of the controlateral ventricular system, the presence of a right frontal-parietal hyper-dense area.

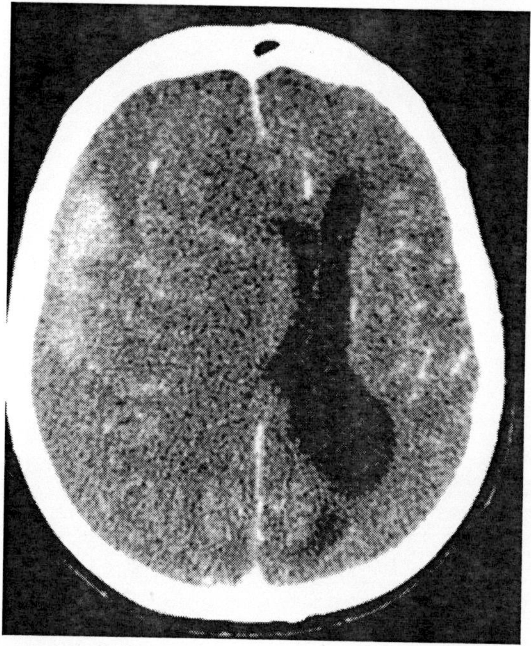

Figure 41. The same case, cerebral CT image after the administration of a contrast substance; the limits of the right hemispheric subdural hematoma are clearly revealed, with the aspect of a two-time hemorrhage.

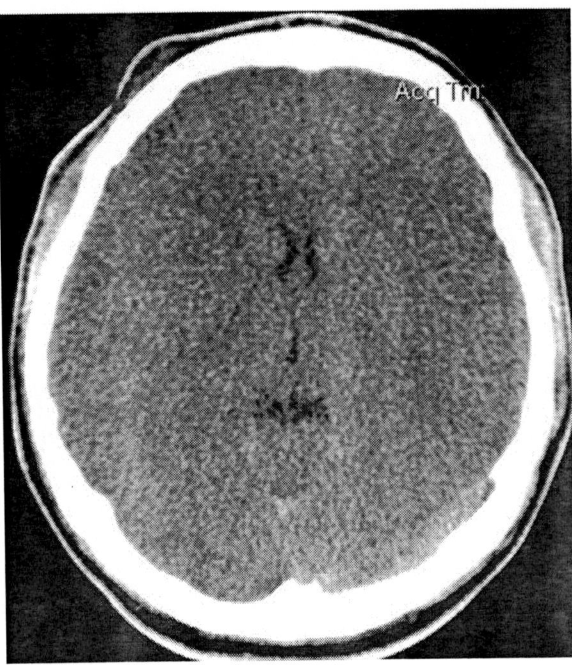

Figure 42. Severe cranial-cerebral traumatism, 3rd degree coma, Glasgow score = 4- 5, cerebral CT: diffuse, bilateral brain edema, compressed perimesencephalic cisterns, with small ventricular system, without focal lesions, Marshall classification: lesional type III; it is a diffuse axonal lesion, type II.

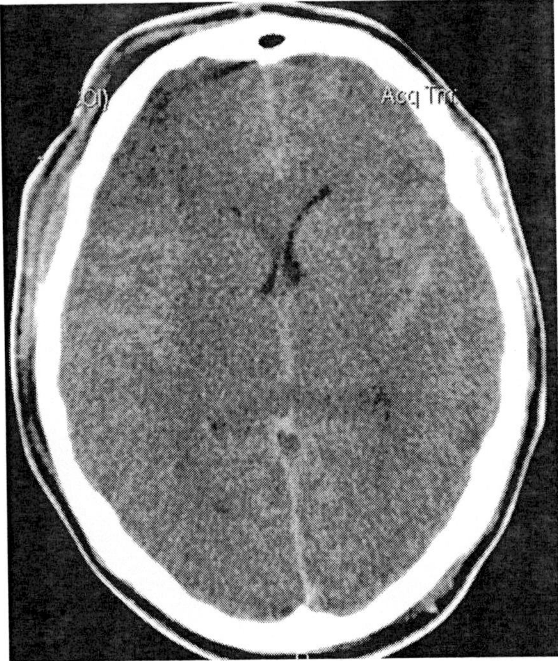

Figure 43. Patient in a 3rd-4th degree coma, with GCS = 4; the CT examination reveals the bilateral diffuse brain edema, the absence of the distinction between the white and gray matter, the small ventricular system, with collapsed peri-mesencephalic cisterns; sub-arachnoid hemorrhage.

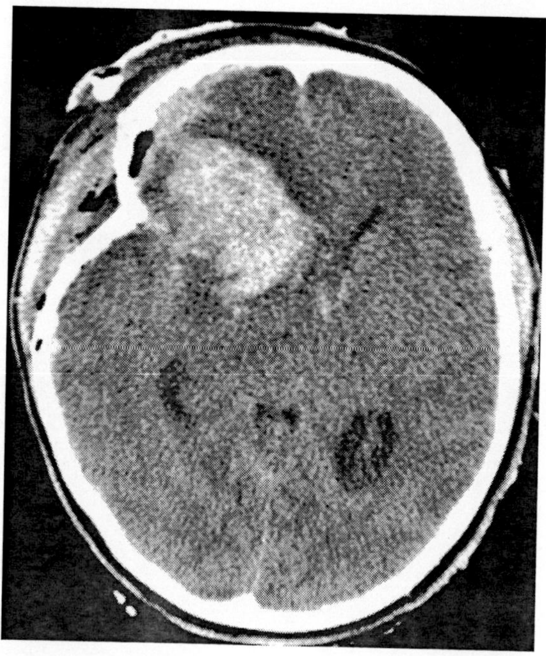

Figure 44. Right intrusive frontal fracture with a focus of contusion – subjacent dilaceration and brain edema with the movement of the ventricular system, which is collapsed. Acute traumatic ICH syndrome, Glasgow score 4

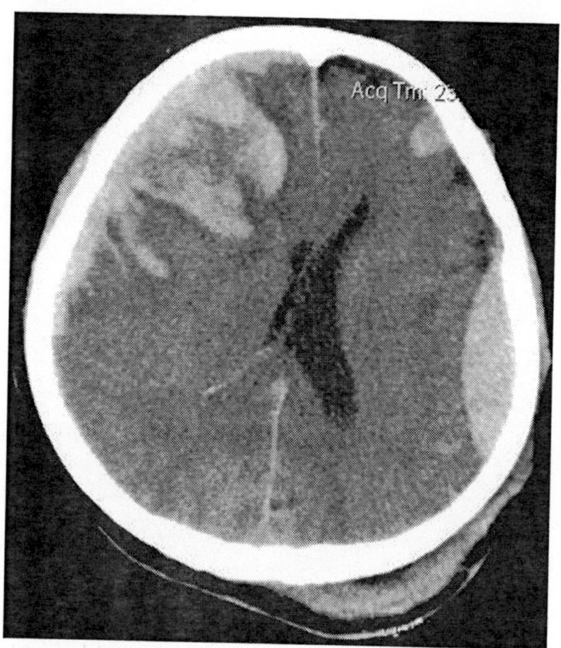

Figure 45. Right frontal contusion with right frontal hematic collection and left hemispheric extradural hematoma. The right hemispheric lesion causes the movement to the left; patient in a 3rd degree coma, Glasgow score 5.

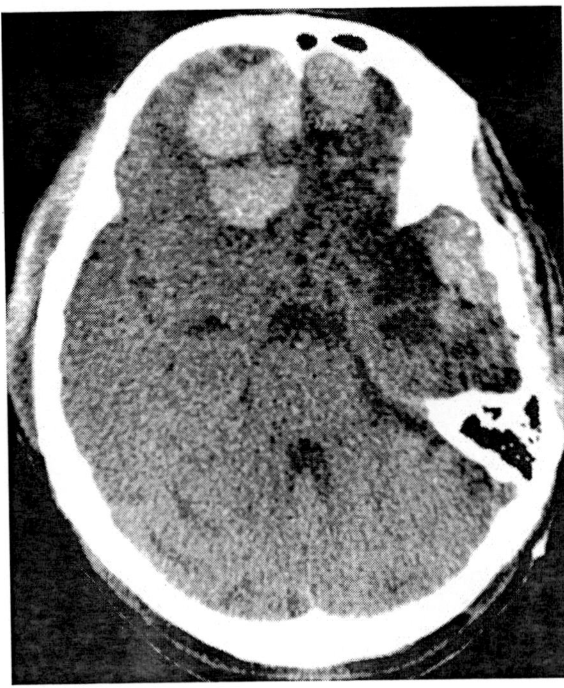

Figure 46. Multiple focuses of cerebral contusion, with acute ICH traumatic syndrome, 2nd degree coma, Glasgow score 6.

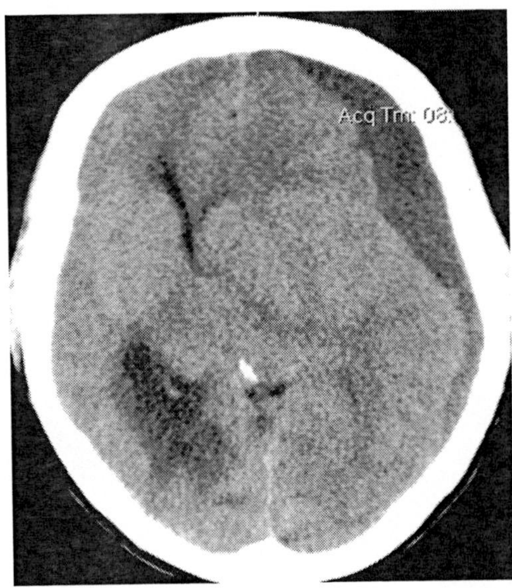

Figure 47. Decompensated chronic subdural hematoma with great controlateral movement of ventricular system, 2nd degree coma, Glasgow score 6.

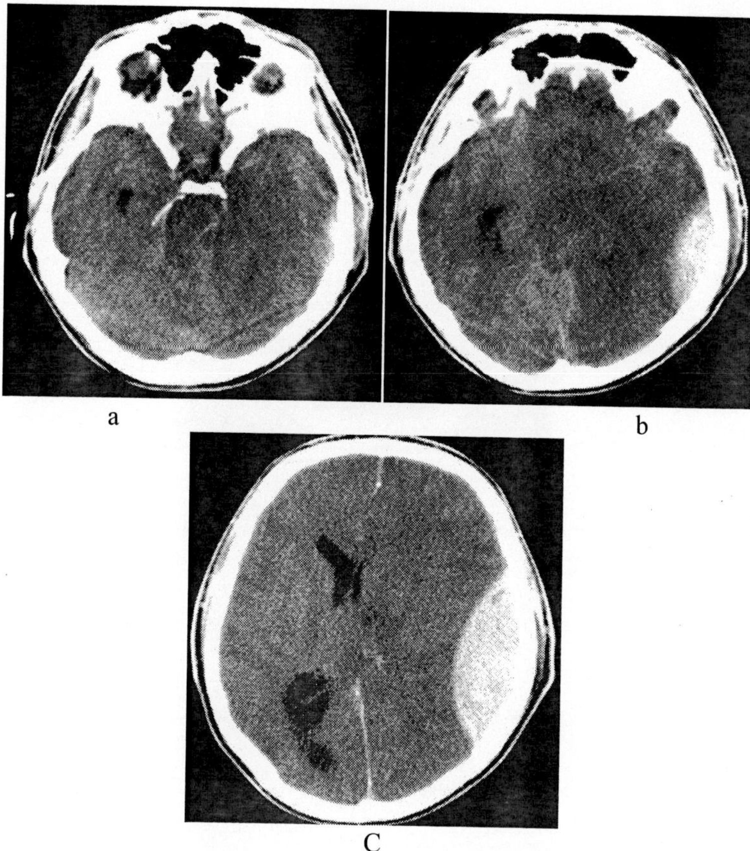

Figure 48. Computer tomography images in the case of a patient with left hemispheric extradural hematoma, with a median line movement, and left temporal herniation with compression and brainstem movement (a)

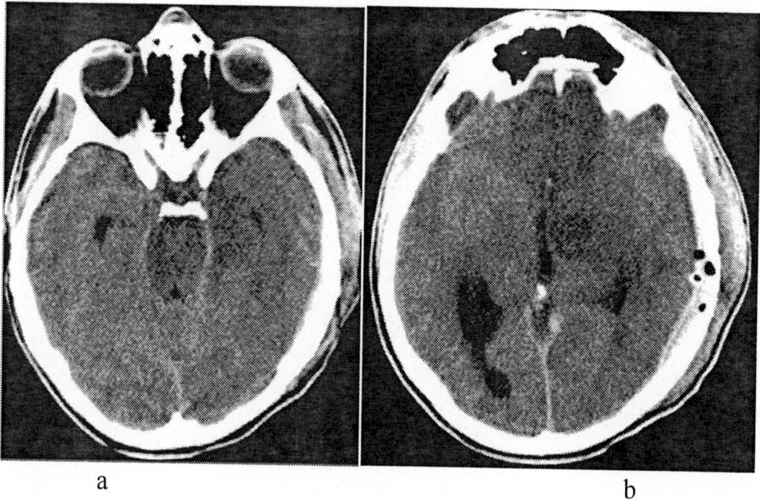

Figure 49. Continues on next page.

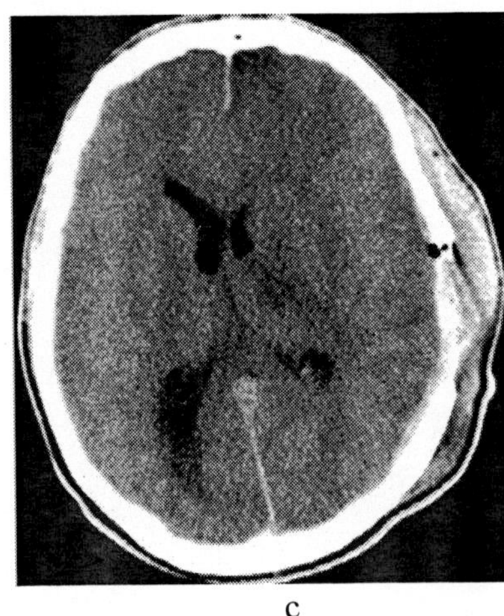

c

Figure 49. Post-surgery computer tomography images of the same patient with left hemispheric extradural hematoma: complete evacuation of the intracranial hematic collection, with a reduced movement of the median axis and a reduced compression of the brainstem, but with diencephalic ischemia and a brainstem ischemia

Magnetic Resonance Imaging

It is superior to the cerebral computer tomography exploration for lesions at the level of the posterior cerebral fossa and in the case of the diffuse axonal lesion. The hemorrhagic cerebral lesions and the diffuse axonal lesions are better identified by nuclear magnetic resonance, but the bone lesions are better identified by a computer tomography. [20,21]

The comparison between these two explorations shows that approximately a quarter of the patients suffering from traumatic brain injury with normal cerebral CT exploration have shown lesions that are identified by means of magnetic resonance.

In the case of severe traumatic brain injury, the magnetic resonance exploration is less recommended in the first moments because of the prolonged duration of the exploration, or often times the patient's vital medical devices, with their metallic components, do not allow the exploration.

Management and Treatment

In the case of a patient with a suspicion of an acute syndrome of traumatic intracranial hypertension, there is an assessment of the consciousness level, the state of conscience, as well as a monitoring of pupil aspect (the patient is examined and the Glasgow score is established). In the case of a patient in coma, the vital conditions are verified (ABC resuscitation succession): free aerial ways, respiration and the circulation function, and the resuscitation maneuvers are executed if needed, with oro-tracheal intubation, etc. Before the radiological information of a cervical lesion, a cervical spinal immobilization is applied. One should also consider the fact that the patient with a severe cranial-cerebral traumatism may be a politraumatized one, which imposes the identification of the vital risk lesions of other organs that require an immediate solution. [1,7,10]

The establishment of the diagnosis and of the management is based on the emergency paraclinical exploration (first of all, the CT scan).

Based on the diagnosis identified by the performed explorations, the cranial-cerebral lesion is evaluated and the optimal option is decided:

- the patient's surgery includes the removal of the pathological supplementary volume with a compressive effect and / or of the cerebral focal lesion that has induced the brain edema. The intracranial pressure decrease is thus ensured and the physio-pathological circuit producing secondary lesions may be interrupted.
- the lesion is diffuse and with no surgical recommendations. The non-surgical focal lesions (which do not produce a compressive effect and / or which have not caused a brain edema before the exploration), the multiple lesions and the diffuse lesions do not benefit from the surgical therapy that may solve the intracranial pressure increase or may stop the secondary lesion progression. In these cases, the therapy is pathogenic with the same purpose of decreasing the intracranial pressure and stopping the secondary lesion evolution.

The traumatic coma without intracranial hypertension requires the pathogenic treatment of the diffuse axonal lesion. [11,14,19]

In the situation of an extremely rapid posttraumatic increase in the intracranial pressure, the immediate effects that cause an aggravation may include pushes and movements of the cerebral parenchyma, with cerebral herniation, or the ICP increase does not leave time for the action of the compensating mechanisms. In the case of the progressive increase in the intracranial pressure, the compensating mechanisms lead to changes in the intracranial fluid dynamics that allow the accommodation of the cerebral circulation to increased pressure values. As a consequence of the accelerated increase in the intracranial pressure, vascular lesions are produced, leading to the traumatic brain edema (mixed edema), to the posttraumatic brain swelling and to the focal or sector ischemic disorders of the nervous parenchyma. The evolution of the secondary traumatic lesions, which are initiated the very moment of the traumatism, may lead to the occurrence and decompensation of the intracranial hypertension. [27,29,31]

In order to evaluate the neurological evolution of these patients and in order to prevent the secondary aggravation by the occurrence or the worsening of a traumatic ICH syndrome, the following are needed:

- general and neurological clinical monitoring,
- cerebral imagistic monitoring,
- knowledge of intracranial pressure values
- knowledge of pressure values for cerebral perfusion which ensures the cerebral blood flux and the optimal cerebral metabolism,
- monitoring the general and cerebral biochemical parameters

The clinical studies and the physio-pathological research have not clarified the controversy whether the increased intracranial pressure or the decreased cerebral perfusion pressure represents the main aggravating factor in severe traumatic brain injury. The purpose of the treatment in severe traumatic brain injury is the normalization of the pathological elements that determine an unfavorable prognosis and the distinction between these two prognosis factors is very important.

If it is considered that the increased intracranial pressure is the most important aggravating factor in the evolution of severe brain trauma, the purpose of the therapy is, first of all, to decrease the increased intracranial pressure, and secondly to improve the cerebral circulation.

If it is considered that the decrease in the cerebral perfusion pressure is the determining aggravating factor, the main purpose of the applied treatment is to maintain the cerebral blood circulation at an adequate level. The maintenance of an appropriate cerebral perfusion imposes therapeutic measures that may lead to the increase in the intracranial pressure. [20,27,31,34]

One may appreciate that, the moment when the brain lesion is produced, the intracranial pressure increase caused by the occurrence of a supplementary intracranial volume is the main aggravating factor, and then the occurrence of cerebral blood circulation disorders are the elements that determine the unfavorable development.

In the case of focal lesions with surgical indications or in the case of multiple focal lesions, the rapid increase in the intracranial pressure seems to be the one causing the worsening, while, in the case of diffuse lesions, the disimprovement is caused by the cerebral circulatory disorders. The decrease in the cerebral perfusion pressure occurs through several mechanisms, and it can be both secondary to the intracranial pressure increase, or it may occur without any relation to the variations of intracranial pressure or in conditions of normal intracranial pressure. [10,20,38]

Therefore, after the surgical solution of the traumatic lesion replacing the intracranial space, which is a solution for the intracranial pressure increase with an immediately posttraumatic occurrence, the therapy continues to be complex, requiring an individualized assessment for every patient as far as the main indication is concerned: to decrease the intracranial pressure or to increase the cerebral perfusion pressure by increasing the systemic arterial pressure, etc., or to evaluate the correlation between the two goals. [21,38,42,43]

Intracranial Pressure Monitoring

The assessment of the intracranial pressure and its monitoring allow:

- the surveillance of the pressure variations and the evaluation of the therapeutic efficiency
- the calculation of the cerebral perfusion pressure, knowing the values of the average blood pressure,
- assessing the resorption capacity of the cerebrospinal fluid,
- the assessment of the intracranial compensating capacities,
- the knowledge of the intracranial sanguine volume.

The appropriate medical treatment is based on these parameters, allowing the assessment of any event that may require another cranial-cerebral computer tomography exploration in order to identify the occurrence of a surgical complication. [20,22]

The indications for the surveillance of the intracranial pressure are all cases of severe traumatic brain injury:

- patients in traumatic cerebral coma with GCS score of between 3 – 8, with a pathological cranial-cerebral computer tomography image that requires a neurosurgical solution.
- patients in traumatic cerebral coma (GCS score : 3 – 8), with a normal CT examination, but who show one of the following risk factors:
- over 40 years of age,
- uni- or bilateral motor deficit, or a uni- or bilateral motor response of the decerebration / decortication type
- the values of the systolic blood pressure are below 90 mm Hg at presentation.

Usually the intracranial pressure monitoring is not performed in patients who have suffered from a medium or slight cranial-cerebral traumatism, and who have a good clinical condition. An ICP monitoring is assessed as necessary in conscious patients where the CT exploration has revealed a limited intracranial traumatic lesion, with a discrete mass effect, and a neurosurgical one at the moment of the CT exploration, patients who present the possibility of an intracranial pressure increase by due to potential development of open cerebral lesions.

The intracranial pressure monitoring is also recommended for patients with a medium cranial-cerebral traumatism (the GCS score is between 9 – 12) on whom the neurological examination can not be repeated because of sedation or of general anesthesia for another therapeutic operation.

At the same time as assessing the intracranial pressure in these patients, other parameters are monitored too, parameters that underline the pathological modifications at the level of the nervous parenchyma:

- there will be a monitoring of the blood pressure, and the best option is an arterial catheter
- permanent ECG surveillance
- oximetry pulse, in order to establish the oxygen saturation in the arterial blood
- oxygen saturation monitoring in the jugular venous blood, $SjvO_2$,
- permanent electroencephalography,
- trans-cranial Doppler ultrasound for cerebral circulation monitoring: intracranial blood flux and speed
- intensive neuro-therapy departments also use: cerebral biochemical findings by micro-dialysis catheters and the calculation of the cerebral oxygen saturation by spectroscopy, Swann-Ganz catheter in the pulmonary artery, etc.

The therapy of severe traumatic brain injury must be based on the data obtained this way, which draw attention on the intracranial pressure increase, the decrease in the cerebral perfusion pressure, at the same time as the treatment of the metabolic disorders in the cerebral parenchyma.

The intracranial pressure must not exceed 20 mm Hg for short periods, of only a few minutes, while prolonged increases require a treatment that would reduce ICP. The interpretation of the intracranial pressure increases is based on the clinical data, which are also correlated to the values of the cerebral perfusion pressure.

A single course of action has not yet been decided on in the assessment of the maximum accepted ICP values a patient with a severe traumatic brain injury: some neuro-reanimation centers consider the maximum limit at which the ICP decreasing treatment is started to be 15 mm Hg, while in other centers, the ICP decreasing therapy begins at values of 25 mmHg; most authors believe that the value of 20 mm Hg is the threshold value at which the intracranial pressure must be decreased. The interpretation of the intracranial pressure values and the necessary treatment must be made based on the clinical development and on the values of the cerebral perfusion pressure. The cerebral perfusion pressure must be maintained at values of over 70 mm Hg, without causing a supplementary increase in the intracranial pressure. [20,21,22]

The care provided to patients with severe traumatic brain injury and the monitoring of their evolution in intensive care and neurosurgery services have established several therapeutic stages, which are recommended depending on the cerebral lesion, on the values of the intracranial pressure, on the need to maintain the cerebral perfusion pressure within normal limits and to prevent secondary cerebral lesions.

Goals:

- removal of primary compressive and/or edematous lesions,
- limiting the edematous effects and/or the cerebral circulation disorders in case of primary lesions,
- prevention, prompt identification and treatment of intracranial and/or systemic pathological disorders that can aggravate the cerebral lesion. The delayed cerebral hemorrhage, the brain edema and the brain swelling are intracranial causes of secondary aggravation, while the arterial hypotension, hypoxia and hyperthermia are systemic causes that lead to the aggravation of the initial lesions.

The Stages of the Intracranial Pressure Monitoring:

1. Installation of the intracranial pressure measuring device and the assessment of the initial values.

In the case of a patient who has undergone a surgery and requires the ICP monitoring immediately after the resolution of the neurosurgical lesion that has caused the acute intracranial hypertension, the normal intracranial pressure values are monitored, as well as the improvement of the cerebral circulation.

If the cerebral perfusion pressure is below 70 mm Hg, the treatment for the correction of the intracranial blood contribution is started, even if ICP is still increased.

If the intracranial pressure has values below 20 mm Hg and the cerebral perfusion pressure is over 70 mm Hg, the patient is supervised, watching the evolution of the ICP and PCP values.

If the intracranial pressure is over 20 mm Hg, the patient is sedated if agitated, and the permeability of the respiratory tracts is checked; moreover, the head is raised at 15 – 25 degrees from horizontal. It is considered that a moderate ICP decrease may be achieved by raising the head. The ICP normalization after these maneuvers does not require other therapeutic actions as far as the intracranial pressure is concerned.

In the case of a patient who does not have a lesion with a surgical indication, but who has an ICP monitoring indication, one must monitor and correct the intracranial pressure increases and the decreases in the cerebral perfusion pressure. ICP values of more than 20 mm Hg require the sedation of an agitated patient and the verification of the respiratory tract permeability. Reduced values of the cerebral perfusion pressure require a specific therapy to maintain the cerebral circulation within normal limits.

2. Immediate monitoring of intracranial pressure values:

- in the case of a patient who has undergone a surgery for a lesion causing acute intracranial hypertension, the ICP decrease occurs because the supplementary volume has been evacuated or there has been a removal of the lesion producing the brain edema, while the craniectomy has turned the cranial cavity into an open room. Due to the evacuation of the supplementary volume (usually a hematoma), ICP decreases in approximately half of the cases; when the brain edematous lesion is removed, the decrease in the brain edema that existed before the neurosurgical intervention is a gradual one, with possible pressure variations that have impacts on the cerebral perfusion.

In almost half of the operated cases, most often in cases of patients with severe cerebral lesions, the preexistent brain edema does not give way once the brain edematous lesion is surgically removed. Although the craniectomy may allow the parenchymatous expansion secondary to the brain edema and then the gradual remission of the edema under an appropriate treatment, the brain edema is seldom diminished and the intracranial pressure is maintained at increased values. The persistent post-surgery intracranial hypertension may be produced by the persistence of the diffuse brain edema, by the progressive extension of the cerebral contusion focuses accompanied by a brain edema, by the hematoma reoccurrence or if certain systemic complications appear.

The values of the intracranial pressure are assessed in correlation to the data provided by the repeated neurological examination. If ICP does not return to normal values and the maintenance of the same neurological condition or a post-surgery neurological degradation are noticed, the cerebral computer tomography is required, in order to reveal an incompletely evacuated lesion, the extension of the preexistent cerebral contusion, the occurrence of a secondary brain edema or the occurrence of secondary ischemic lesions.

The specific therapy is required in these circumstances: a new surgical intervention, perhaps with an enlarged craniectomy with a decompressive effect or the cerebral vascular vasodilating and anti-spastic treatment.

If the new cerebral CT exploration does not reveal a lesion with surgery indication, but the intracranial pressure is maintained at high values, a set of therapeutic measure are progressively applied, measures that may be schematized based on their therapeutic efficiency.

Treatment Scheme in Case of Intracranial Pressure Increase

The objectives of the treatment are:

- maintaining ICP within normal limits, at values below 20 mm Hg, and
- maintaining an appropriate cerebral perfusion pressure, above 70 mm Hg.

Depending on the intracranial pressure value and on PCP, the ICP decreasing therapy or the therapy for the correction of the cerebral perfusion is applied, or the patient is monitored.

The therapy aiming to decrease the ICP increases and maintain PCP within normal limits is applied gradually, depending on the ICP and PCP monitoring values and on the other parameters, establishing three therapeutic stages. If the therapeutic measures are efficient, this therapeutic stage is not ended, and the patient continues to be monitored; but, if the intracranial pressure does not decrease, the following therapeutic measures are applied. [2,3,4,6,8]

First Therapeutic Measures or 1st Degree (First Line) Measures:

I. Sedation and perhaps a moderate hyper-ventilation
This is applied as long as ICP < 20 mm Hg for the first 12 hours.

- sedatives
- $PaCO_2$ is maintained at ≈ 35 mm Hg, in the case of mechanically ventilated patients

If the ICP value is higher than 20 mm Hg, one must check whether the increased pressure values are due to the patient's agitation or if there is a mechanical obstruction that may lead to the pressure increase. The patient who manifests a psycho-motor agitation is sedated and, if ICP decreases below 20 mm Hg, the surveillance is continued, as well as the pathogenic and symptomatic therapy at the intensive care department.

II. The cerebrospinal fluid drainage. If ICP $>$ 19 - 20 mm Hg for more than 5 minutes, the cerebrospinal fluid drainage is used whenever needed, as long as the operation is an efficient one.

III. Use of diuretics

If ICP is maintained increased over 20 mm Hg for more than 5 minutes, the following may be used:

- osmotic diuretics: mannitol administration.
- loop diuretics: furosemide is used

The combination of these two diuretics is more efficient and it requires the monitoring of the blood electrolytes (potassium). [9,11,12,13,16]

Therapeutic Measures Of 2nd Degree (2nd Line):

IV. Hyperventilation, hypothermia concomitantly with a hypertensive therapy

- controlled hypothermia with the maintenance of a temperature of 34 – 35 ° C.
- hypertensive therapy for the increase in the systemic blood pressure in order to ensure a normal cerebral perfusion pressure in the conditions of an increased ICP; in the case of a cerebral contusion, the systemic arterial pressure is increased to 150 – 170 mm Hg, and, if there is no cerebral contusion, the blood pressure may increase up to 180 mm Hg.
- hyperventilation, which leads to $PaCO_2$ of 25 – 30 mm Hg. Hyperventilation generates a cerebral vasoconstriction, and ICP decreases by the decrease in the cerebral blood flux. Hyperventilation is intermittent, and it is not recommended on the first day after a severe cranial-cerebral traumatism.[9,19,23,24,25]

V. Administration of a NaCl hypertonic solution, concentration of 7.5 %.

VI. Surgical decompression: the cerebral CT exploration excludes the development of a new compressive intracranial lesion, the brain edema is very important, and the performance of a large decompressive unilateral or bilateral craniectomy is considered.

VII. The anesthetic therapy is performed under the electroencephalographic control to doses that diminish the EEG activity:

- non-barbituric hypnotic substances: etomidate, propofol.
- barbituric substances: phenobarbital, thiopental (barbituric coma).

Third degree therapeutic measures (3rd line),

are used in exceptional cases:

VIII. Trometamol (THAM) decreases the partial CO_2 pressure and causes a cerebral vasoconstriction, only if the cerebral vessel reactivity to CO_2 is intact.

IX. The cerebrospinal drainage by lumbar puncture is applied after the exhaustion of the other therapeutic means if the cerebral computer tomography exploration reveals the presence of the basal cisterns and the non-collapsed lateral ventricles. In this case, the risk of a brain herniation produced by this operation, *which is usually not recommended in ICH*, is lower than the possibility of an unfavorable evolution due to the worsening of the intracranial pressure increase. [26,28,30,32,36,37,39,40,41]

A. Non-traumatic acute parenchymatous intracranial hypertension

The parenchymatous intracranial hypertension with an acute start may occur in non-traumatic parenchymatous intracranial lesions with a sudden start such as the intra-parenchymatous hematomas occurred on the background of the high blood pressureor by the break of a cerebral vascular malformation, etc. Often, in these situations, the brutal increase in the volume of the intra-cerebral hematoma is combined with the blockage of the cerebrospinal fluid circulation by the blood effraction in the ventricular system, which also generates the occurrence of an acute obstructive hydrocephalus.

The parenchymatous intracranial hypertension with an acute start may also occur in the case of an apparently asymptomatic intracranial lesion, with a compensated ICH syndrome, by the sudden surpassing of the pressure compensating mechanisms. This is the acute clinical manifestation of the decompensation of the parenchymatous intracranial hypertension with a progressive start. [10,15,18]

In the case of intracranial tumors, with post-surgery irradiation, or radio-surgical procedures have been applied (gamma knife), there may be a significant increase in the tumor volume, of up to 30%, which generates acute phenomena of intracranial hypertension.

The clinical presentationis the one of the acute intracranial hypertension syndrome, and it includes:

- preexistent symptoms greatly and rapidly accentuated: cephalea, vomiting, psychic disorders, etc.;
- initial convulsive crises or preexistent crises with increased frequency and duration;
- worsening or occurrence of the pyramidal syndrome, cranial nerves palsy;
- consciousness disorders and coma.

The clinics of the ICH syndrome aggravation has been classically presented by Cushing: bradycardia, increase in the systemic blood pressure and the occurrence of respiratory disorders. The occurrence of the unilateral mydriasis represents an alarm signal for the temporal cerebral herniation.

The rapidly performed paraclinical explorations establish the existence of an intracranial expansive process that requires a surgical solution for the removal of the supplementary endocranial volume.

The parenchymatous intracranial hypertension with an acute start may also occur in the absence of an intracranial space replacing lesion in the case of the posterior reversible encephalopathy syndrome (PRES) [also designated as the reversible posterior leuco-encephalopathy syndrome = RPLS] of non-hypertensive etiology. The posterior reversible encephalopathy syndrome (PRES) is the clinical manifestation of an acute, reversible ICH syndrome.

The clinical presentation is a typical one: cephalea, vomiting, conscience disorders, convulsive crises, visual disorders, and it may occur in two situations:

- acute high blodd pressure episode: in renal conditions, eclampsia; it is included in vascular ICH.
- administration of immuno-suppressors or cytostatics.

The pathogenic parenchymatous mechanism consists of the neurotoxic action of immuno-suppressors and cytostatics, with the production of a vasoconstriction followed by the cerebral hypo-perfusion and the occurrence of the brain ischemia with the development of the cytotoxic brain edema.

The CT or MRI imaging is characteristic: brain edema with a posterior bilateral location, with sub-cortical interest of the white matter, while the DWI emphasizes the cellular brain edema by decreased water mobility.

The treatment consists of stopping the immuno-suppressing or cytostatics medication with gradual improvement in a few days.

The parenchymatous intracranial hypertension with an acute start of toxic cause may occur in the fulminating case of hepatic failure. In the cases of fulminating hepatic failure, the etiology of the intracranial hypertension is represented by the cytotoxic brain edema due to the astrocyte accumulation of glutamine and the vasogenic brain edema due to the disruption of the blood-brain barrier; there is also an increase in the cerebral blood volume and in cerebral blood flow, partly due to inflammation, to glutamine and to toxic products of the diseased liver. In the fulminating hepatic insufficiency with acute ICH, the neurological prognosis may be established by determining the ICP, and it is extremely important because it allows the decision of a hepatic transplant to be made.

II. Progressive Parenchymatous Intracranial Hypertension

General Data

Intracranial expansive processes with a progressive development can have the initial clinical manifestation of a neurological focus syndrome or by a non-specific symptomatology, to which the symptomatology of the intracranial hypertension is gradually added afterwards.

Depending on the location and the development manner, intracranial expansive processes cause the progressive increase in the intracranial pressure and then the occurrence of the ICH syndrome by the development of a supplementary volume. [18,20,21,35,38]

The new endocranial volume may be represented by:

- the lesion that replaces the intracranial space (endocranial tumor, intra-parenchymatous hematoma, subdural chronic hematoma, cerebral abscess, etc.), whose volume has increased progressively;

- the secondary brain edema of a primary lesion having a relatively reduced volume; extended brain edema with a compressive effect on the fluid spaces and on adjacent parenchymatous structures.

Benign intracranial tumors have a slow volume increasing rate and the neurological syndrome is installed progressively, while the ICH syndrome may occur late.

Malignant tumors have a rapid development rate and the neurological syndrome occurs precociously.

The clinical decompensation represents the aggravation of the symptomatology by the tumor extension or by exceeding the compensating capacities of the intracranial pressure increase, and it manifests itself by:

- increase in the frequency of comitial crises,
- occurrence or accentuation of neurological deficits,
- occurrence of symptoms and installation of the ICH syndrome,
- occurrence of consciousness disorders: confusion syndrome, apathy, etc.
- installation of coma.

The occurrence of the intracranial hypertension syndrome depends on the characteristics of the endocranial lesions. These lesion characteristics refer to:

- the speed of the increase in the supplementary endocranial volume, which depends on the nature of the lesion (benign or malignant tumor, intra-cerebral hematoma, subdural chronic hematoma, etc.):
- benign tumor lesions have a slow increase, with moderate cerebral suffering,
- the sudden occurrence of the intracranial hypertension may suggest a rapid expansion at the level of the tumor by producing an intra-tumor hemorrhage or the accelerated development of a tumor cyst
- the biological effect on the adjacent cerebral tissue (direct, compressive edematous effect, etc.):
- malignant gliomas lead to the occurrence of the brain edema, they produce neoformation vessels, etc.
- cerebral metastases are accompanied by an important brain edema and the intracranial hypertension is frequently present.
- the location of the supplementary volume (direct compression on the vital structures, blockage of the cerebrospinal fluid circulation):
- subtentorial tumors evolve more frequently with ICH compared to supratentorial tumors, because the circulation of the cerebrospinal fluid may be blocked by the peritumoral edema and by the location of the tumor,
- tumors, even the malignant ones localized at the frontal, occipital pole, can develop for long periods of time with no ICH syndrome.

The period that includes the changes in the intracranial pressure, reaching and then exceeding the normal pressure limit values is long, with a slow increasing speed of the intracranial pressure, and decompensation can take place rapidly or after a longer period of time. During the infraclinical period, there is a compensation of the pressure increases caused by the newly added volume, but the limit pressure is reached. Once the compensating capacities are exceeded, the intracranial pressure increase is rapid, and the duration of these pathological pressure values is short due to the rapid decompensation.

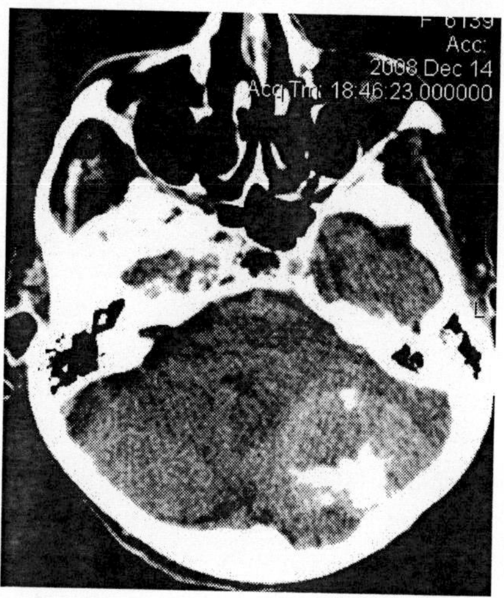

Figure 50. Subtentorial tumor with blocked fourth ventricle.

There is also the possibility of a slow increase in intracranial pressure: with a prolonged infraclinical period and a long period of pathologic ICP increase. The ICP increases slowly and progressively up to the normal limit value, and it continues its slow increase depending on the ICH etiology. The ability to compensate the pressure increase allows a prolonged maintenance of the cerebral blood flux, and there is a long period of the pathological pressure values. The ICH syndrome is prolonged and its aggravation is rapidly produced, surpassing all the compensating methods of pressure increases.

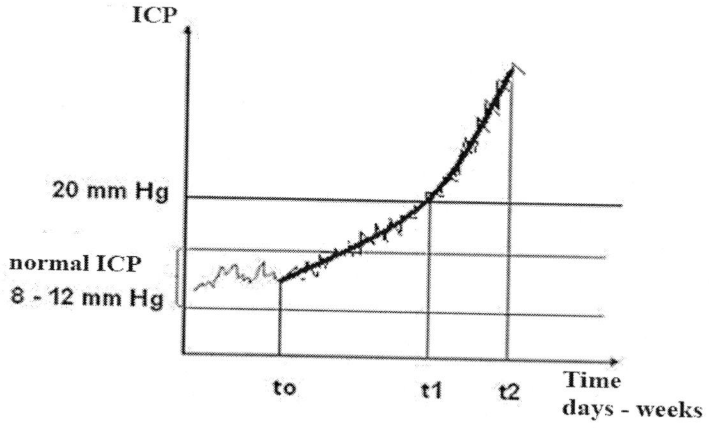

Figure 51. Acute ICP increase, with a prolonged infraclinical period and a rapid decompensation; the interval to-t1 is prolonged, weeks or even months, and the decompensation may last for a few days.

Low-grade Gliomas

They are cerebral tumors with a slow increasing rate, most frequently they have a supratentorial location, especially frontal and temporal, or they may be developed in the brainstem, and they are more frequent in young adults.

The dominating symptoms are motor deficient, epileptic crises, cephalea and psychic disorders.

The ICH syndrome with a papillary edema occurs more rarely because the location does not affect the circulation of the cerebrospinal fluid and because the dominating symptoms bring the patient to the physician before the increase in the tumor volume, which produces signs of intracranial hypertension.

High-grade Gliomas

They are malignant cerebral tumors, usually located deep into the white matter, but sometimes they may also have an intra-ventricular development or, from the deep cerebral hemispheric white matter, they may have a cortical extension.

The mechanisms that lead to the occurrence of the symptomatology are:

- local parenchymatous effects:
  - compression on the neighbouring structures: nervous parenchyma, cerebral vessels or the circulation paths of the cerebrospinal fluid,
  - the tumor invasion on the neighbouring structures: nervous parenchyma and/or cerebral vessels,
  - local tissue destruction with the formation of the cellular degrading products,
  - hypoxia of the neighbouring nervous tissue by the direct compression of the blood vessels too,
  - metabolic and electrolytic disorders
  - release of cytokines, of free radicals, etc.
- diffuse intracranial effects caused by:
  - the increase in the intracranial pressure by
    - the tumor volume
    - the secondary effects of the volume increase on the cerebral parenchyma, on the blood circulation and on the dynamics of the cerebrospinal fluid.

The symptomatology is:

- focal neurological syndromes:
  - irritation syndrome: psychic disorders, epileptic crises

- syndrome in a deficit: sensitive or motor.
- syndrome of progressive intracranial hypertension:
  - psychic disorders,
  - cephalea,
  - vomiting,
  - papillary edema, etc.

Brain Metastases

Cerebral metastases are accompanied by an important brain edema, and intracranial hypertension is frequently present. The single cerebral metastasis may be focalized anywhere in the cerebral parenchyma and it practically has the characteristics of a malign cerebral tumor; multiple metastases usually exceed the direct surgical therapeutic possibilities.

The symptomatology depends on the location of the lesion/lesions and on the occurrence of the intracranial hypertension through well-known mechanisms.

Intra-Cerebral Hematoma

In the primary intra-cerebral hematomas, the occurrence and development of the intracranial hypertension depends on preexistent factors (elements of hypertensive encephalopathy), on the volume of the hematoma and on the superficial or deep lumbar location, in the oval center, on the communication with the ventricular system, and perhaps on the circulating blockage of the cerebrospinal fluid.

Chronic Subdural Hematoma

The chronic subdural hematoma is a well-known neurosurgical entity; it occurs after a usually minor cranial traumatism, and it is characterized by the slow evolution of the "pre-clinical" period.

Usually, the focal neurological symptomatology is of a first ground interest, but, sometimes, the ICH syndrome may be marked, especially in the case of a brain trauma, which subsequently produces clinical decompensation.

Benign Intracranial Tumors

Benign intracranial tumors are represented by meningiomas, neurinomas, pituitary tumors, etc. The benign intracranial tumors present a slow increasing rate, and the symptomatology is represented by the focal neurological syndromes, and, usually at a delayed stage, by the intracranial hypertension syndrome. They most frequently cause the occurrence of the ICH syndrome by blocking the circulation of the cerebrospinal fluid, producing an intracranial hypertension by disorders of the cerebrospinal fluid dynamics. Secondly, the benign intracranial tumor induces a peritumoral brain edema, which brings about the occurrence of a parenchymatous intracranial hypertension with a progressive evolution.

Other Endocranial Lesions

Other types of expansive intracranial lesions – cerebral abscesses, dural empyemas, parasitoses (hydatid cyst), etc., present variable evolutions of the intracranial hypertension syndrome based on the same characteristics: location of the lesion, the expansion speed and the edematous character of lesions.

The Relationship between Lesion Location and ICH Occurrence

In the case of a parenchymatous ICH with a gradual start, the relation between the location of the lesion and the occurrence of the intracranial hypertension syndrome seems less significant because the blocking mechanism of the cerebrospinal fluid circulation with the ICH occurrence by the compressive lesion of the ventricular system, belongs to the intracranial hypertension by disorders of the cerebrospinal fluid dynamics.

The multiple concomitant regional monitoring of the intracranial pressure has revealed the existence of significant pressure differences between the values of the sector intracranial pressure, especially in the case of temporal lesions, which may evolve towards decompensation by cerebral hernia before the ICP equalization in all the endocranial compartments.

Usually, the occurrence and rapid decompensation of the intracranial hypertension, which is explained by the location of the lesion, frames this type in the ICH by blocking the circulation of the cerebrospinal fluid and by the occurrence of the acute obstructive hydrocephalus.

References

[1] Adamides AA, Winter CD, Lewis PM, Cooper DJ, Kossmann T, Rosenfeld JV.Current controversies in the management of patients with severe traumatic brain injury.*ANZ J.* Surg. 2006 ;76(3):163-74.

[2] Albanese J, Leone M, Alliez JR, Kaya JM, Antonini F, Alliez B, Martin C. Decompressive craniectomy for severe traumatic brain injury: Evaluation of the effects at one year. *Crit. Care Med.* 2003.;31(10): 2535-8.

[3] Allan R, Chaseling R. Subtemporal decompression for slit-ventricle syndrome: successful outcome after dramatic change in intracranial pressure wave morphology. Report of two cases. *J. Neurosurg.* 2004 ;101(Suppl):214-7.

[4] Ayr LK, Yeates KO, Taylor HG, Browne M. Dimensions of postconcussive symptoms in children with mild traumatic brain injuries. *J. Int. Neuropsychol. Soc.*2009 ;15(1):19-30.

[5] Balestreri M, Steiner LA, Czosnyka M. Sex-related differences and traumatic brain injury. *J. Neurosurg.* 2003 99(3):616 .

[6] Bedford RF, Morris L, Jane JA. Intracranial hypertension during surgery for supratentorial tumor: correlation with preoperative computed tomography scans. *Anesth. Analg.* 1982 ; 61(5):430-3.

[7] Bell MJ, Kochanek PM. Traumatic brain injury in children: recent advances in management.*Indian J. Pediatr.* 2008 Nov;75(11):1159-65.

[8] Berger S, Schwarz M, Huth R. Hypertonic saline solution and decompressive craniectomy for treatment of intracranial hypertension in pediatric severe traumatic brain injury. *J. Trauma.* 2002 ; 53(3):558-63.

[9] Caricato A, Conti G, Della Corte F, Mancino A,et al Effects of PEEP on the intracranial system of patients with head injury and subarachnoid hemorrhage: the role of respiratory system compliance. *J. Trauma.* 2005 ;58(3):571-6.

[10] Ciurea AV, Nuteanu L, Simionescu N, Georgescu S. Posterior fossa extradural hematomas in children: report of nine cases. *Childs Nerv. Syst.* 1993 ;9(4):224-8.

[11] Cruz J, Minoja G, Okuchi K. Major clinical and physiological benefits of early high doses of mannitol for intraparenchymal temporal lobe hemorrhages with abnormal pupillary widening: a randomized trial. *Neurosurgery.* 2002 ;51(3):628-37.

[12] Dziedzic T, Szczudlik A, Klimkowicz A, Rog TM, Slowik A. Is mannitol safe for patients with intracerebral hemorrhages? Renal considerations.*Clin. Neur. Neurosurg.* 2003 ;105(2):87-9.

[13] Figaji AA, Fieggen AG, Peter JC. Early decompressive craniotomy in children with severe traumatic brain injury.*Childs Nerv. Syst.* 2003 ;19(9):666-73.

[14] Flierl MA, Smith WR, Morgan SJ, Stahel PF. Molecular mechanisms and management of traumatic brain injury - missing the link? *World J. Emerg. Surg.* 2009 4;4:10.

[15] Fritsch MJ, Doerner L, Kienke S, Mehdorn HM. Hydrocephalus in children with posterior fossa tumors: role of endoscopic third ventriculostomy. *J. Neurosurg.* 2005;103(1 Suppl):40-2

[16] Grande PO, Naredi S. Clinical studies in severe traumatic brain injury: a controversial issue. *Intensive Care Med.* 2002 ;28(5):529-31

[17] He XS, Zhang X. Giant calcified chronic subdural haematoma: a long term complication of shunted hydrocephalus.*J. Neurol. Neurosurg. Psychiatry.* 2005 ;76(3):367.

[18] Hlatky R, Valadka AB, Robertson CS. Intracranial hypertension and cerebral ischemia after severe traumatic brain injury. *Neurosurg .Focus.* 2003 ,15;14(4):e2.

[19] Huang WD, Pan J, Xu M, Su W et al Changes and effects of plasma arginine vasopressin in traumatic brain injury. J Endocrinol Invest. 2008 ;31(11):996-1000.

[20] Iencean St M A new classification and a synergetical pattern in intracranial hypertension *Medical Hypotheses* , 2002 ;58(2):159-63.

[21] Iencean St M Pattern of increased intracranial pressure and classification of intracranial hypertension. *Journal of Medical Sciences,* 2004, vol.4,Nr.1 :52- 58

[22] Iencean St M Classification and essential conditions of decompensation in intracranial hypertension *Rom. J. Neurosurgery* 2004, 1 ;1,. 3-13

[23] Inenaga C, Tanaka T, Sakai N, et al: Diagnostic and surgical strategies for intractable spontaneous intracranial hypotension. Case report. J Neurosurg 94:642–645, 2001

[24] Kamat P, Vats A, Gross M, Checchia PA. Use of hypertonic saline for the treatment of altered mental status associated with diabetic ketoacidosis. *Pediatr. Crit Care Med.* 2003 ;4(2):239-42.

[25] Kontopoulos V, Foroglou N et al Decompressive craniectomy for the management of patients with refractory hypertension: should it be reconsidered? *Acta Neurochir.* (Wien). 2002 ; 144 (8):791-6.

[26] Marcoux KK. Management of increased intracranial pressure in the critically ill child with an acute neurological injury. *AACN Clin Issues.* 2005 ;16(2):212-31.

[27] Mathew P, Teasdale G, Bannan A, Oluoch-Olunya D. Neurosurgical management of cerebellar haematoma and infarct. J Neurol Neurosurg Psychiatry. 1995; 59: 287–292.

[28] Mori K, Ishimaru S, Maeda M. Unco-parahippocampectomy for direct surgical treatment of downward transtentorial herniation. *Acta Neurochir.* 1998; 140: 1239–1244.

[29] Mowery NT, Gunter OL, Guillamondegui O et al Stress insulin resistance is a marker for mortality in traumatic brain injury. *J. Trauma.* 2009 ;66(1):145-51;

[30] Mussack T, Huber SM, Ladurner R, Hummel T, Mutschler W. Bilateral decompressive craniectomy due to intracranial hypertension during acute posttraumatic liver dysfunction. *J. Trauma.* 2005 ;58(5):1061-5.

[31] Owler BK, Besser M. Extradural hematoma causing venous sinus obstruction and pseudotumor cerebri syndrome. *Childs Nerv. Syst.* 2005 ;21(3):262-4.

[32] Psarros TG, Coimbra C. Endoscopic third ventriculostomy for patients with hydrocephalus and fourth ventricular cysticercosis: a review of five cases. *Minim Invasive Neurosurg.* 2004 ; 47(6):346-9.

[33] Roberts I, Schierhout G, Wakai A. Mannitol for acute traumatic brain injury. *Cochrane Database Syst Rev.* 2003;(2):CD001049. Review.

[34] Salim A, Hadjizacharia P, Dubose J et al Persistent hyperglycemia in severe traumatic brain injury: an independent predictor of outcome.*Am. Surg.* 2009 ;75(1):25-9.

[35] Scarone P, Losa M, Mortini P, Giovanelli M. Obstructive Hydrocephalus and Intracranial Hypertension Caused by a Giant Macroprolactinoma. Prompt Response to Medical Treatment. *J. Neurooncol.* 2006 ;76(1):51-4.

[36] Schneider GH, Bardt T, Lanksch WR, Unterberg A. Decompressive craniectomy following traumatic brain injury: ICP, CPP and neurological outcome. *Acta Neurochir. Suppl.* 2002;81:77

[37] Shiozaki T, Nakajima Y, Taneda M, etc all. Efficacy of moderate hypothermia in patients with severe head injury and intracranial hypertension refractory to mild hypothermia. *J. Neurosurg.* 2003 ;99(1):47-51.

[38] Soffietti R, Ruda R, Mutani R. Management of brain metastases.*J. Neurol.*2002; 249(10):1357

[39] Steiner LA, Balestreri M, Johnston AJ, Coles JP,et al Predicting the response of intracranial pressure to moderate hyperventilation. *Acta Neurochir.* (Wien). 2005; 147(5):477-83.

[40] Vincent JL, Berre J. Primer on medical management of severe brain injury. *Crit Care Med.* 2005 ;33(6):1392-9.

[41] Watling CJ, Cairncross JG. Acetazolamide therapy for symptomatic plateau waves in patients with brain tumors. Report of three cases. *J. Neurosurg.* 2002 ;97(1):224-6.

[42] Winter CD, Adamides AA, Lewis PM, Rosenfeld JV. A review of the current management of severe traumatic brain injury.*Surgeon*. 2005 ;3(5):329-37.

[43] Winter CD, Adamides A, Rosenfeld JV.The role of decompressive craniectomy in the management of traumatic brain injury: a critical review.*J. Clin. Neurosci.* 2005 ; 12(6):619-23.

Chapter XI

Vascular Intracranial Hypertension

General Data

Intracranial hypertension can occur in cerebral-vascular illnesses due to blood cerebral or extra-cerebral circulatory disorders, which modify the dynamics of the intracranial fluids and cause the intracranial pressure increase. There are disorders in the auto-regulation of the cerebral hemodynamics and the cerebral parenchyma volume continues to increase due to the brain edema or to the increase in the cerebral sanguine volume (brain swelling) with the secondary increase in the intracranial pressure. [4,15,26]

The volume of the cerebral parenchyma increases due to the modifications occurred at the level of the cerebral sanguine capillaries, which leads to:

- the occurrence of the extracellular brain edema due to the increased quantity of interstitial fluid:
    - extracellular edema produced by a hydrostatic mechanism (ultra-filtration) in severe arterial hypertension,
    - extracellular edema with oncotic induction (vasogenic edema) due to an increased permeability of the brain blood barrier (open brain-blood barrier)
- brain swelling with an increase in the volume of the cerebral parenchyma by vascular dilatation.

The vascular types of intracranial hypertension have characteristic etiologies and they occur by:

- slowing down or decreasing the intracranial venous flux in thrombophlebites and cerebral venous thrombosis, the decrease in the venous flux at the level of the superior longitudinal sinus (SLS) directly in compressive lesions (hollowing fracture, etc.) or in SLS shunting by an intracranial arterial-venous malformation, or the extra-cranial illnesses that block the returning venous circulation at the cervical level, reduce the cerebral venous drainage and cause the decrease in the absorption of the cranial-spinal fluid and then the occurrence of the brain edema.

- in hypertensive encephalopathy, when the hydrostatic brain edema occurs (by ultra-filtration), as well as a brain swelling (by vasodilatation).
- the cerebral ischemia or the ischemic stroke reduces the arterial blood input and causes an ischemic brain edema, which is a mixed brain edema, both a cellular edema (cytotoxic) and an extracellular brain edema with oncotic induction (vasogenic). [26,27,46,49]

Cerebral Venous Thrombosis

The cerebral venous drainage is slowed-down or even stopped in illnesses that influence the intracranial venous circulation or on extra-cranial conditions that may interest the great vessels at the level of the throat, usually by compression from vicinity. [5,6,7,8,26]

The cerebral venous circulation is reduced in:

- cerebral thrombophlebites and superficial venous thrombosis,
- thrombosis of dural sinuses,
- thrombosis of the profound venous system, and
- thrombosis of the cavernous sinus. [11,12,16]

The thrombotic venous occlusion is more frequent in the following etiological situations:

- infections (usually, the local infections are: otitis, sinusitis, etc., also in the case of meningitis). Mastoiditis may produce the thrombosis of the venous sinuses with a syndrome of secondary intracranial hypertension, an entity that Symonds describes as “otitic hydrocephalus”,
- tumor lesions at the level of the sinus, with its infiltration and obstruction (especially in meningiomas), when the tumor development is not responsible for the occurrence of ICH,
- traumatic brain injury,
- pregnancy and puerperium, etc.
- the calcifications of the sinus extended scythe have a reduced incidence (Figure 53).

The frequency of the impacts on the dural sinuses and of other cerebral veins is as follows:

- the thrombosis of the sagittal sinus and of the lateral sinuses is happens in 75 – 85 % of cases
- the thrombosis of the superficial cortical veins occurs in approximately 10 – 15 % of cases,
- the thrombosis of the profound cerebral veins occurs in approximately 5 – 10 % of cases, and
- the thrombosis of the cavernous sinus occurs in less than 5 % of cases.

Cerebral venous thrombosis reduce the returning venous circulation from the brain and the skull, a venous stasis is produced and the cerebral circulation is slowed down. There are areas of cerebral hypo-anorexia concomitantly to areas of venous swelling, and the cellular cerebral (cytotoxic) edema occurs, as well as the oncotic extracellular (vasogenic) edema, which evolves to a mixed brain edema. [20,21,22,32,33]

The venous sinuses also ensure the resorption of the cerebrospinal fluid, and the thrombosis of the venous sinuses leads to a diminished drainage of the cerebrospinal fluid. Therefore, a progressive intra-ventricular accumulation of cerebrospinal fluid occurs, with a pressure increase in the ventricular system and the occurrence of the hydrocephalic brain edema.

These phenomena happen slowly, in varied successions, but the evolution is progressive towards an intracranial pressure increase.

The iatrogenic thrombosis of the internal jugular veins is quoted in cases of prolonged use of the jugular catheters for the intravenous administration of medication. In such cases, the same pathogenic processes occur, and the ICH syndrome may appear.

The symptomatology is caused by the initial causal lesion, after which neurological focal symptoms may occur related to the progression of the venous thrombosis, as well as symptoms caused by the intracranial pressure increase. A venous infarct often happens, which is associated to a cerebral hemorrhage, which also aggravates the neurological clinical presentation.

Usually, the clinic condition evolves to an incomplete or complete syndrome of intracranial hypertension. [34,37,39,41,42,52]

The main characteristics of the intracranial pressure increase in cerebral venous thrombosis are:

- a slow increase in the intracranial pressure up to the normal limit value of 20 mm Hg, usually during a period of a few days,
- over the value of 20 mm Hg, the ICP increase continues to be progressive, and it may reach maximum values of approximately 30 – 40 mm Hg in a few hours or days. This gradual increase allows the compensating mechanisms to act more efficiently, and also for the applied therapy to encourage the intracranial pressure decrease and the improvement of the cerebral circulation.
- the maximum values that may be reached in cases of intracranial hypertension syndrome are of approximately 30- 35 mm Hg (sometimes the maximum values may be of 40 mm Hg) and
- the pathological pressure values may last for several weeks, with a slow return to normal pressure values and period of intermittent increases,
- usually, there is a recurrence to intracranial pressure values of about and above 20 mm Hg, which causes the persistency of a prolonged attenuated symptomatology.

The treatment of the venous thrombosis with an ICH syndrome is as follows:

- etiological and pathogenic for the vascular disorder, when possible,
- pathogenic for the intracranial hypertension syndrome.

A particular pathogenic mechanism is the reduction of the venous flux at the level of the superior longitudinal sinus (SLS) with an important blockage of the cerebrospinal fluid resorption:

- in aneurysm of the vein of Galen when there is a superior sagittal sinus shunting by malformation and the cerebrospinal fluid resorption is diminished by the occurrence of the hydrocephalus. In infants and small children, the dominating symptomatology is the cardiac disorder due to the increased venous return, while the ICH syndrome also occurs in older children.
- in the case of a median depressed skull fracture which interests the third posterior part of the superior sagittal sinus.
- at children with craniostenosis, there may be anomalies of the venous drainage, which interests the sigmoid sinus and the jugular vein, which may cause a venous hypertension, with a diminished drainage of the cerebrospinal fluid and the increase in the intracranial pressure. Usually, the phenomenon occurs up to the age of 6 years old, after which a collateral venous drainage is developed by the stylomastoid plexus, leading to the normalization of the intracranial pressure.

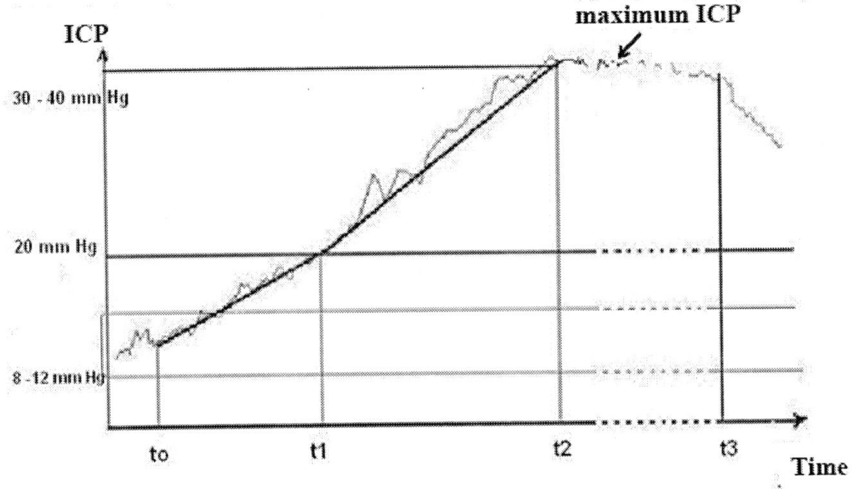

Figure 52 . Cranial pressure increase in cerebral venous thrombosis:

- to = start of the cerebral venous thrombosis
- t1 = the moment when the normal limit value of 20 mm Hg is reached
- t2 = after the progressive increase in the intracranial pressure, the maximum values of approximately 30 – 35 mm Hg are reached
- t3 = the moment when, after a varied period of increased pressure values, the ICP begins to decrease progressively, usually after treatment

Δ t1 = t1 – to : the period of intracranial pressure increase up to the normal limit value of 20 mm Hg, which usually lasts for a few days

Δ t2 = t2 – t1 : the ICP increase period up to the maximum value, which may last for several hours to several days

Δ t3 = t3 – t2 : the period of time of maximum intracranial pressure values, which usually last for several weeks.

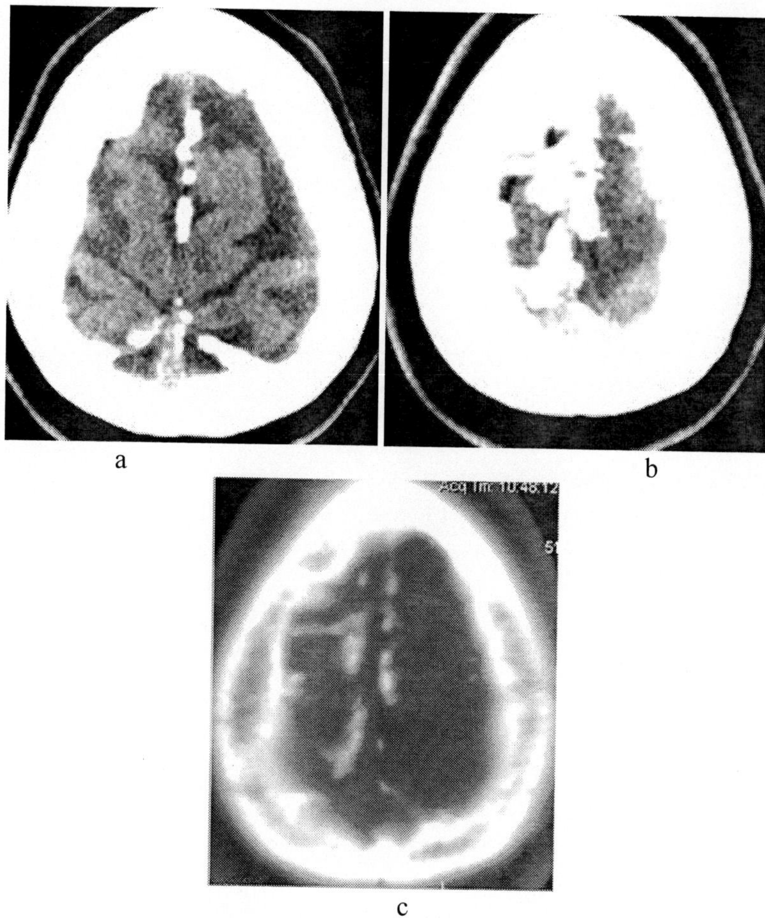

Figure 53. Calcifications at the level of the brain scythe (a), extended towards the superior longitudinal sinus (b), bilateral (c), with a slowing-down of the venous drainage, a decreased resorption of the cerebrospinal fluid and an ICH syndrome.

Hypertensive Encephalopathy

High blood pressure is the most important predisposing factor for cerebrovascular illnesses, and the most frequent complication is the cerebral hemorrhage. The exaggerated increase in the values of the systemic blood pressure also causes disorders of the cerebral circulation auto-regulation, with other secondary cerebral suffering.

Hypertensive encephalopathy is defined in the clinical presentationof induced intracranial hypertension by an acute episode of arterial hypertension. [4,15,26]

1. The acute hypertensive encephalopathy is caused by the acute blood pressure increase in:

- severe high blood pressure,
- uncontrolled / untreated high blood pressure in pregnancy (eclampsia),
- high blood pressure in glomerulonephritis, pheochromocytoma, etc.

The acute increase in the sanguine pressure values leads to the inefficiency of the cerebral vascular auto-regulation, a generalized cerebral vascular dilatation occurs and / or there is an increased permeability of the cerebral capillaries. The increased permeability in the brain blood barrier has been constant more frequently at the level of the gray matter.

Therefore, the increase in the volume of the cerebral parenchyma is caused by:

- brain swelling by vasodilatation,
- hydrostatic extracellular brain edema, by ultra-filtration when the brain blood barrier is intact (close brain-blood barrier)
- oncotic (vasogenic) extracellular brain edema by an injury of the brain blood barrier (open brain-blood barrier).

The posterior reversible encephalopathy syndrome (PRES) or the reversible posterior leuco-encephalopathy syndrome (RPLS) with a hypertensive etiology is included in the acute form of vascular etiopathogeny ICH. The clinical presentation is typical and the DWI exploration shows an extracellular brain edema by the increase in the water mobility with a posterior bilateral location and a sub-cortical interest in the white matter too. The treatment consists of decreasing the systemic blood pressure. [26,27,31,53]

2. The chronic hypertensive encephalopathy (Binswanger encephalopathy) is a rare cerebrovascular illness with a chronic extracellular brain edema: hydrostatic brain edema combined with the oncotic brain edema.

The ICP increase in acute hypertensive encephalopathies are characterized by:

- the relatively high speed with which the intracranial pressure reaches the normal threshold value in approximately a few hours
- the ICP continues to increase above the normal values for a period that is usually shorter than the previous interval, of few hours only
- the maximum values that the ICP may reach are of 30 – 50 mm Hg and
- the period with pathologic intracranial pressure values is usually of several hours, rarely of several days. The anti-hypertensive treatment improves the clinical condition.
- The unmonitored hypertensive patients, or those who are incompletely treated may present repeated episodes of hypertensive encephalopathy, or they may suffer from the most frequent complication, which is the cerebral hemorrhage.

The clinical evolution of hypertensive encephalopathy is up to an incomplete syndrome of intracranial hypertension, and it has a regressive aspect. In the pathogeny of the syndrome, there is an auto-limiting mechanism: the intracranial pressure increase caused by the increase in the blood pressure and by occurrence of the cerebral vasodilatation generated the collapse of the walls of the intracranial vessels, and, to a certain extent, to a diminished cerebral blood volume. The mechanism consists of the direct action of the increased intracranial pressure over a functional disorder that is secondary to the exceeded auto-regulation of the cerebral circulation, and it has a limited value.

The treatment of the hypertensive encephalopathy is both etiologic and pathogenic:

- the treatment of the hypertensive episode, as an etiologic aspect, and
- the pathogenic treatment of the intracranial hypertension syndrome

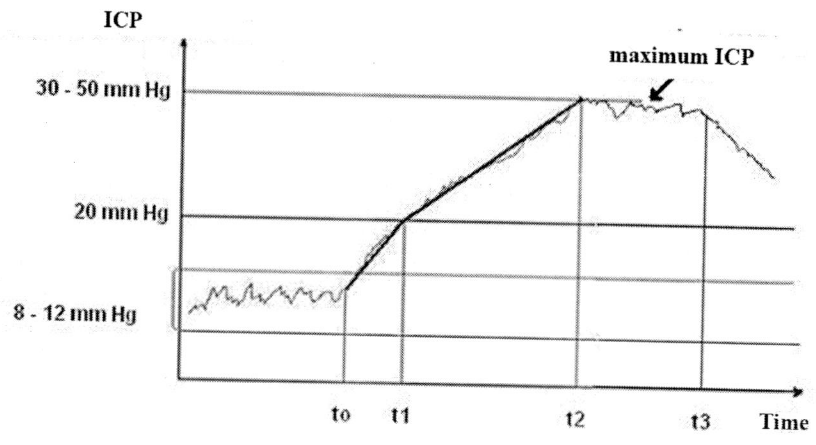

Figure 54. Intracranial pressure increase in hypertensive encephalopathy:
to = beginning of the increase in the sanguine blood pressure
t1 = the moment when the normal ICP limit value is reached
t2 = the moment when the ICP has the maximum value
t3 = beginning of the decrease in the intracranial pressure values
Δ t1 = t1 – to : period of ICP increase up to the normal limit; it lasts for several hours
Δ t2 = t2 – t1 : the ICP increase period to the maximum values, lasting for several hours
Δ t3 = t3 – t2 : the period when the pathologic ICP values are maintained, usually of a few hours; it is rarely prolonged to a few days; the causal treatment of the high blood pressureis efficient.

Ischaemic Stroke

The cerebral ischemia is caused by the cerebral circulatory insufficiency, which may be chronic or acute. [1,2,3,9,11]

The acute cerebral circulatory insufficiency or the ischemic stroke can manifest itself as:

- transitory ischemic stroke,
- progressive ischemic stroke,
- regressive ischemic stroke,
- complete ischemic stroke or the cerebral infarction. The cerebral infarction can be of a thrombotic or embolic origin.

The ischemic stroke represents 85 % of the cerebrovascular illnesses. The large ischemic cerebral lesions are accompanied by the brain edema with cerebral herniation (sub-falciform) and by the intracranial pressure increase. [13,14,15,17]

There are multiple causes of the ischemic cerebral vascular stroke:

- vascular illnesses: carotid atherosclerosis, infectious arteriopathies, posttraumatic occlusions of internal carotid arteries, of vertebral arteries or of middle cerebral arteries, arterial compressions at the cervical level, various vasculopathies,
- cerebral embolism of a cardiac cause – which represents approximately 60 - 70 % of the cerebral embolism cases: in the case of a mitral illness with atrial fibrillation, coronary thrombosis, paradoxical embolisms, infectious endocardites, etc.
- there may be rare cases of: hyper-coagulability, policitemia vera, etc.

The extended cerebral ischemic infarction with phenomena of intracranial hypertension is caused by the occlusion or stenosis of a great cerebral artery: the internal carotid artery or a terminal branch that irrigates a vast territory, such as the middle cerebral artery.

The total ischemic infarction of the Sylvian artery occurs in approximately 10 % of the patients with acute cerebral circulatory insufficiency, and it has been designated as the malignant infarction of the middle cerebral artery (MCA = Sylvian artery) due to the increased mortality, of up to 80 % of cases, despite the therapeutic means used. [1,17,18,19,24,25]

The massive cerebellum ischemic infarction can cause the collapse of the 4th ventricle with the occurrence of an acute obstructive hydrocephalus and an acute ICH syndrome, and it has a direct compressive effect on the brainstem with the manifestation of vegetative disorders.

In the case of the cerebral hemispheric ischemic stroke, the decreased blood flow in the territory of the middle cerebral artery leads to the occurrence of certain ischemic metabolic disorders at the level of the affected cerebral parenchyma. The permeability of the cerebral capillaries increases (open brain-blood barrier) and the extracellular oncotic (vasogenic) edema occurs. The evolution is usually a rapid one, with the extension of the brain edema, the increase in the intracranial pressure and the occurrence of the sub-falciform cerebral hernia (median line movement towards the unaffected cerebral hemisphere). Although the intracranial pressure increasing mechanism is based on the cerebral ischemia with a hypoxic brain edema, which is characteristic for the parenchymatous lesions, while the etiology is represented by the impacts on a great cerebral artery, and it includes the ischemic stroke on vascular intracranial hypertension. [26,28,29,30,35]

Since the moment of the arterial occlusion, the intracranial pressure increase is:

- rapid until it reaches the normal pressure limit of 20 mm Hg, by the progression of the brain edema and the surpassing of the pressure compensating possibilities, with a duration of up to several hours
- above the normal pressure values, the ICP increase is also a rapid one, and the maximum values are reached within a short interval of time: half an hour – several hours
- the maximum values of the intracranial pressure are of approximately 40 – 50 mm Hg and
- the duration of these pathological values is of several days and it corresponds to the intensive care period.

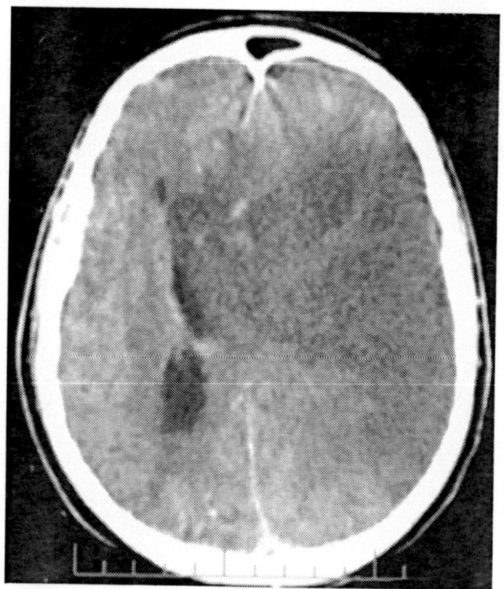

Figure 55. Malignant infarct ion of left Sylvian artery with important ischemic brain edema and sub-falciform cerebral herniation (cardiac rhythm disorder) .

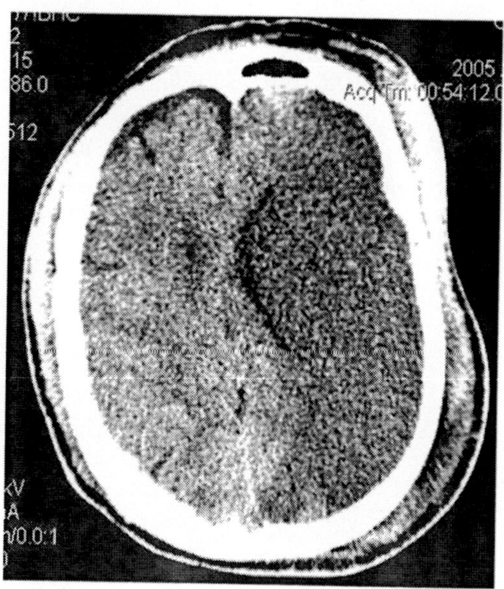

Figure 56 Complete infarction of left MCA (traumatic occlusion at the level of the throat - strangulation)

The evolution is rapid towards the decompensation of the intracranial hypertension with almost 80% unfavorable results despite the applied treatments.

There is an attempt in using the etiological treatment of the arterial obstruction and the pathogenic treatment for the ICH syndrome. During the first three hours from the beginning, there may be an intravenous administration of recombined tissue plasminogen activator (rtPA) in a dose of 0.9 mg/kg, maximum 90 mg; the administration of streptokinase or of other thrombolytic agents does not have the same efficiency as rtPA. The brain edema receives a pathogenic treatment with osmotic diuretics (mannitol), and hyperventilation if there is an imminent decompensation of intracranial hypertension and the production of a brain herniation etc. [1,35,36,38,40,43,47]

Sometimes, there is an attempt of a surgical intervention:

- decompressive craniectomy of posterior cerebral fosse and of evacuation of a cerebellum infarction with a compressive effect on the brainstem, perhaps with a ventricular drainage,
- decompressive craniectomy and the evacuation of a cerebral hemispheric massive infarction, which may diminish the intracranial hypertension, but the surviving patients is left with major neurological deficits.

A particular case of generalized cerebral ischemia is met in the post-resuscitation syndrome when the sanguine flux disorder includes the entire brain, with a complete ischemia throughout the stroke, followed by reperfusion disorders.[26,48,50,51,54,55]

The consequence of this cerebral circulatory failure, primary – before and during cardiopulmonary resuscitation, and secondary ischemic damage, during reperfusion is the development of the mixed brain edema: both cytotoxic and vasogenic, concomitantly to the production of the glial and neuronal necrosis. The hyperemic reperfusion may exacerbate the brain edema.

The mixed brain edema accentuates the elevated intracranial pressure and it exacerbates the brain injury.

The treatment is complex and the results do not compensate the efforts.

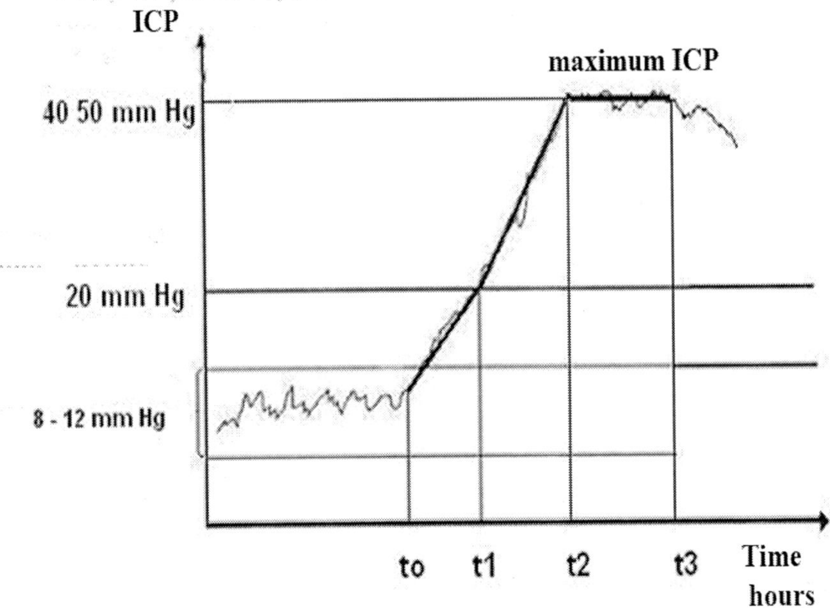

Figure 57. Characteristics of the intracranial pressure increase in the ischemic stroke:

to = the moment when the arterial occlusion happens

t1 = the moment when the normal ICP limit value is reached

t2 = the moment when the ICP value is at maximum, of approximately 40 –50 mm Hg

t3 = the moment when the ICP begins to decrease; the ICP value diminishing is rare in the Sylvian malignant ischemic stroke

Δ t1 = t1 – to : the ICP increasing period up to the maximum normal value; it lasts for several hours

Δ t2 = t2 – t1 : the period when ICP reaches the maximum values, lasting for a half an hour – one hour

Δ t3 = t3 – t2 : the period when the pathological ICP values are maintained; it may last for several days.

The table below includes a comparative presentation of the three forms of vascular intracranial hypertension.

Table 3. Etio-pathogenic and evolutionary characteristics of the various forms of vascular ICH

Cerebral venous thrombosis	Hypertensive encephalopathy	Ischemic stroke
Cerebral vascular pathology: - thrombosis of dural sinuses - thrombosis of cortical veins	Cerebral vascular pathology: - dilatation of cerebral arteries	Cerebral vascular pathology: - infarct of Sylvian artery - massive cerebellum infarct
Cerebral blood flow : Reduced venous outflow	Cerebral blood flow : Increase arterial inflow	Cerebral blood flow : Reduced arterial inflow
Pathogenesis: - venous dilatation; open BBB and vasogenic brain edema and - diminished CSF drainage with hydrocephalic brain edema	Pathogenesis: - dilatation of cerebral vessels; closed BBB and hydrostatic brain edema, and -increased vascular permeability with open BBB and vasogenic brain edema	Pathogenesis: - ischemic increased capillary permeability ; open BBB and vasogenic brain edema
ICP increase: - slow to the normal limit - slow above the normal limit	ICP increase: - rapid to the normal limit - slow above the normal limit	ICP increase: - rapid to the normal limit - rapid above the normal limit
Sub-acute and chronic evolution Possible decompensation	Acute and sub-acute evolution Rarely decompensation	Acute evolution Usually decompensation
Pathogenic treatment	Pathogenic and etiologic treatment	Etiologic and pathogenic treatment, Decompressive craniectomy

References

[1] Albers GW, Bates VE, Clark WM, Bell R, Verro P, Hamilton SA. Intravenous tissue-type plasminogen activator for treatment of acute stroke: the Standard Treatment with Alteplase to Reverse Stroke (STARS) study. *JAMA.* 2000; 283: 1145–1150.

[2] Alberts MJ, Hademenos G, Latchaw RE, et al. Recommendations for the establishment of primary stroke centers: Brain Attack Coalition. *JAMA.* 2001; 283: 3102–3109.

[3] Asil T, Uzunca I, Utku U, Berberoglu U. Monitoring of increased intracranial pressure resulting from cerebral edema with transcranial Doppler sonography in patients with middle cerebral artery infarction. *J. Ultrasound Med.* 2003 ;22(10):1049-53

[4] Bateman GA. Vascular hydraulics associated with idiopathic and secondary intracranial hypertension. *Am. J. Neuroradiol.* 2002 ;23(7):1180-6.

[5] Bergui M, Bradac GB. Clinical picture of patients with cerebral venous thrombosis and patterns of dural sinus involvement. *Cerebrovasc. Dis.* 2003;16(3):211-6.

[6] Biousse V, Tong F, Newman NJ. Cerebral Venous Thrombosis. *Curr. Treat. Options. Neurol.* 2003 ;5 (5):409-420.

[7] Brandt T, Pessin MS, Kwan ES, Caplan LR. Survival with basilar artery occlusion. *Cerebrovasc Dis.* 1995; 5: 182–187.

[8] Brandt T, von Kummer R, Muller-Kuppers M, Hacke W. Thrombolytic therapy of acute basilar artery occlusion: variables affecting recanalization and outcome. *Stroke.* 1996; 27: 875–881.

[9] Brott T, Bogousslavsky J. Treatment of acute ischemic stroke. *N. Engl. J. Med.* 2000; 343: 710–722.

[10] Brown MM. Surgical decompression of patients with large middle cerebral artery infarcts is effective: not proven. *Stroke.* 2003 ;34(9):2305-6.

[11] Carter BS, Ogilvy CS, Candia GJ, Rosas HD, Buonanno F. One-year outcome after decompressive surgery for massive nondominant hemispheric infarction. *Neurosurgery.* 1997; 40: 1168–1175.

[12] Chopko BW, Kerber C, Wong W, Georgy B. Transcatheter snare removal of acute middle cerebral artery thromboembolism: technical case report. *Neurosurgery.* 2000; 40: 1529–1531.

[13] Christou I, Alexandrov AV, Burgin WS, et al. Timing of recanalization after tissue plasminogen activator therapy determined by transcranial doppler correlates with clinical recovery from ischemic stroke. *Stroke.* 2000; 31: 1812–1816.

[14] Coull BM, Williams LS, Goldstein LB, et al. Anticoagulants and antiplatelet agents in acute ischemic stroke. *Stroke*. 2002; 33: 1934–1942.

[15] Cruz J, Minoja G, Okuchi K. Major clinical and physiological benefits of early high doses of mannitol for intraparenchymal temporal lobe hemorrhages with abnormal pupillary widening: a randomized trial. *Neurosurgery.* 2002 ;51(3):628-37.

[16] Cumurciuc R, Crassard I, Sarov M, Valade D, Bousser MG. Headache as the only neurological sign of cerebral venous thrombosis: a series of 17 cases. *J. Neurol. Neurosurg Psychiatry.* 2005 ; 76(8):1084-7.

[17] Demchuk AM, Burgin WS, Christou I, et al. Thrombolysis in brain ischemia (TIBI) transcranial Doppler flow grades predict clinical severity, early recovery, and mortality in patients treated with intravenous tissue plasminogen activator. *Stroke.* 2001; 32: 89–93.

[18] Demchuk AM, Tanne D, Hill MD, et al. Predictors of good outcome after intravenous tPA for acute ischemic stroke. *Neurology.* 2001; 57: 474–480.

[19] Diener HC, Ringelstein EB, von Kummer R, et al. Treatment of acute ischemic stroke with the low-molecular-weight heparin certoparin: results of the TOPAS trial: Therapy of Patients with Acute Stroke (TOPAS) Investigators. *Stroke.* 2001; 32: 22–29.

[20] Eckstein HH, Schumacher H, Dorfler A, et al. Carotid endarterectomy and intracranial thrombolysis: simultaneous and staged procedures in ischemic stroke. *J. Vasc. Surg.* 1999; 29: 459–471.

[21] Farb RI, Vanek I, Scott JN, Mikulis DJ, Willinsky RA,et al Idiopathic intracranial hypertension: the prevalence and morphology of sinovenous stenosis. *Neurology*. 2003 13;60(9):1418-24.

[22] Ferro JM, Canhao P, Bousser MG, et al Cerebral vein and dural sinus thrombosis in elderly patients. *Stroke.* 2005 ;36(9):1927-32

[23] Ferro JM, Lopes MG, Rosas MJ, et al Delay in hospital admission of patients with cerebral vein and dural sinus thrombosis. *Cerebrovasc Dis.* 2005;19(3):152-6.

[24] Fraser JF, Hartl R. Decompressive craniectomy as a therapeutic option in the treatment of hemispheric stroke. *Curr .Atheroscler. Rep.* 2005 ;7(4):296-304.

[25] Hajat C, Hajat S, Sharma P. Effects of poststroke pyrexia on stroke outcome: a meta-analysis of studies in patients. *Stroke.* 2000; 31: 410–414.

[26] Iencean St M A new classification and a synergetical pattern in intracranial hypertension *Medical Hypotheses* , 2002 ;58(2):159-63.

[27] Iencean St M Vascular intracranial hypertension, *J Med.Sciences* 2004 . 4, 4 : 276 – 281

[28] Jansen O, Schellinger P, Fiebach J, Hacke W, Sartor K. Early recanalisation in acute ischaemic stroke saves tissue at risk defined by MRI. *Lancet.* 1999; 353: 2036–2037.

[29] Kakinuma K, Ezuka I, Takai N, Yamamoto K, Sasaki O. The simple indicator for revascularization of acute middle cerebral artery occlusion using angiogram and ultra-early embolectomy. *Surg. Neurol.* 1999; 51: 332–341.

[30] Kalafut MA, Schriger DL, Saver JL, Starkman S. Detection of early CT signs of >1/3 middle cerebral artery infarctions: interrater reliability and sensitivity of CT interpretation by physicians involved in acute stroke care. *Stroke.* 2000; 31: 1667–1671.

[31] Kanazawa M, Sanpei K, Kasuga K. Recurrent hypertensive brainstem encephalopathy.*J. Neurol. Neurosurg. Psychiatry.* 2005 ;76(6):888-90.

[32] Kasper GC, Wladis AR, Lohr JM, et al. Carotid thromboendarterectomy for recent total occlusion of the internal carotid artery. *J. Vasc. Surg.* 2001; 33: 242–250.

[33] Kidwell CS, Saver JL, Mattiello J, et al. Thrombolytic reversal of acute human cerebral ischemic injury shown by diffusion/perfusion magnetic resonance imaging. *Ann. Neurol.* 2000; 47: 621

[34] King JO, Mitchell PJ, Thomson KR, et al: Cerebral venography and manometry in idiopathic intracranial hypertension. *Neurology*,45:2224–2228, 1995

[35] von Kummer R, Nolte PN, Schnittger H, Thron A, Ringelstein EB. Detectability of cerebral hemisphere ischaemic infarcts by CT within 6 h of stroke. *Neuroradiology.* 1996; 38: 31–33.

[36] Kuo JR, Lin CL, Chio CC, Wang JJ, Lin MT. Effects of hypertonic (3%) saline in rats with circulatory shock and cerebral ischemia after heatstroke. *Int. Care Med.*2003; 29(9):1567-73.

[37] Linskey ME, Sekhar LN, Hecht ST. Emergency embolectomy for embolic occlusion of the middle cerebral artery after internal carotid artery balloon test occlusion: case report. *J. Neurosurg.* 1992; 77: 134–138.

[38] Mathew P, Teasdale G, Bannan A, Oluoch-Olunya D. Neurosurgical management of cerebellar haematoma and infarct. *J Neurol.Neurosurg. Psychiatry.* 1995; 59: 287–292.

[39] McCormick PW, Spetzler RF, Bailes JE et. al Thromboendarterectomy of the symptomatic occluded internal carotid artery. *J. Neurosurg.* 1992; 76: 752–758.

[40] Melgar MA, Rafols J, Gloss D, Diaz FG. Postischemic reperfusion: ultrastructural blood-brain barrier and hemodynamic correlative changes in an awake model of transient forebrain ischemia. *Neurosurgery.* 2005 ;56(3):571-81.

[41] Owler BK, Besser M. Extradural hematoma causing venous sinus obstruction and pseudotumor cerebri syndrome. *Childs Nerv. Syst.* 2005 ;21(3):262-4.

[42] Owler BK, Parker G, Halmagyi GM, Pseudotumor cerebri syndrome: venous sinus obstruction and its treatment with stent placement. *J. Neurosurg.* 2003 ;98(5):1045-55.

[43] Oyelese AA, Steinberg GK, Huhn SL, Wijman CA. Paradoxical cerebral herniation secondary to lumbar puncture after decompressive craniectomy for a large space-occupying hemispheric stroke: case report. *Neurosurgery.* 2005 ;57(3):E594

[44] Phatouros CC, Higashida RT et al. Endovascular stenting of an acutely thrombosed basilar artery: technical case report and review of the literature. *Neurosurgery.* 1999; 44: 667–673.

[45] Rajpal S, Niemann DB, Turk AS. Transverse venous sinus stent placement as treatment for benign intracranial hypertension in a young male: case report and review of the literature. *J. Neurosurg.* 2005 ;102(3 Suppl):342-6.

[46] Santarius T, Menon DK. Images in clinical medicine. Carotid-artery thrombosis secondary to basal skull fracture. *N. Engl. J. Med.* 2003 , 31;349(5):e5.

[47] Schlaug G, Benfield A, Baird AE, et al. The ischemic penumbra: operationally defined by diffusion and perfusion MRI. *Neurology.* 1999; 52: 1528–1537.

[48] Schwab S, Hacke W. Surgical decompression of patients with large middle cerebral artery infarcts is effective. *Stroke.* 2003 ;34(9):2304-5.

[49] Sindou M, Auque J, Jouanneau E. Neurosurgery and the intracranial venous system. *Acta Neurochir. Suppl.* 2005;94:167-75.

[50] Steiger H-J. Outcome of acute supratentorial cerebral infarction in patients under 60: development of a prognostic grading system. *Acta Neurochir.* 1991; 111: 73–79.

[51] Suh DC, Sung KB, Cho YS, et al. Transluminal angioplasty for middle cerebral artery stenosis in patients with acute ischemic stroke. *Am. J. Neuroradiol.* 1999; 20: 553–558.

[52] Tamimi A, Abu-Elrub M, Shudifat A et al . Superior sagittal sinus thrombosis associated with raised intracranial pressure in closed head injury with depressed skull fracture. *Pediatr Neurosurg.* 2005 ;41(5):237-40.

[53] Tsumoto T, Miyamoto T, Shimizu M, et al . Restenosis of the sigmoid sinus after stenting for treatment of intracranial venous hypertension: case report. *Neuroradiology.*2003; 45(12):911-5.

[54] Walters BB, Ojemann RG, Heros RC. Emergency carotid endarterectomy. *J. Neurosurg.* 1987; 66: 817–823.

[55] Yoshimoto Y, Kwak S. Superficial temporal artery-middle cerebral artery anastomosis for acute cerebral ischemia: the effect of small augmentation of blood flow. *Acta Neurochir.* 1995; 137: 128–137.

Chapter XII

Intracranial Hypertension Due to Disorders in the Cerebrospinal Fluid Dynamics

General Data

The intracranial hypertension due to disorders in the cerebrospinal fluid dynamics is the intracranial pressure increase caused by disorders of the cerebrospinal fluid circulation from the moment of its formation at the level of the choroid plexuses and until its passage in the venous circulation. [1,3,11,17,18]

The dynamic disorders of the cerebrospinal fluid are:

- circulation disorders of the cerebrospinal fluid from formation to the resorption place and
- disorders of the cerebrospinal fluid passage in the venous drainage system (resorption).

The circulation disorders of the cerebrospinal fluid are caused by an obstacle along the fluid route (ventricular system, magna cistern, basal cisterns) due to an obstruction by a ventricular or paraventricular tumor, an intra-ventricular hemorrhage or an obstruction due to various causes of the Sylvian aqueduct. The segments of the ventricular systems, which are superjacent to the obstruction, increase their volume, creating an obstructive internal hydrocephalus.

The resorption disorders of the cerebrospinal fluid occur due to the injury of the anatomic structures or due to disorders of the physiological mechanisms that assure the cerebrospinal fluid passage in the drainage venous system. These phenomena occur in acute meningitis, in sub-arachnoid hemorrhage, in meningeal carcinomatosis, in chronic sarcoidosis meningitis, etc. Most frequently there is a thickening of the leptomeninges blocking the Pachioni arachnoid corpuscles and decreasing the cerebrospinal fluid absorption. The cerebrospinal fluid—accumulates in the ventricular system and a communicating hydrocephalus occurs, with a periventricular hydrocephalic brain edema and with a generally sub-acute intracranial hypertension syndrome, designated as meningeal intracranial hypertension. The clinical presentationand the type of intracranial pressure increase resemble the intracranial hypertension syndrome met in the obstruction cases of cerebrospinal fluid circulation. [17,18]

Disorders in Cerebrospinal Fluid Flow and Obstructive Hydrocephalus

The obstructive hydrocephalus is caused by a partial or complete obstruction of the ventricular system or by a blockage of the CSF flow. [1,2,4,5,8]

The ventricular blockage is achieved by:

- stenosis of Sylvian aqueduct – malformation, tumor, by intra-ventricular hemorrhage or inflammatory secondary stenosis.
- expansive intra-ventricular processes of 3rd ventricle or 4th ventricle that block the circulation of the cerebrospinal fluid.
- extrinsic blockage of the ventricular system due to paraventricular lesions. These may be expansive intracranial processes of cranium base, of posterior cerebral fosse, of median line (sellar, parasellar, etc.), which, through local compression and cerebral movement, cause the ventricular obstruction (the 3rd ventricle, Sylvian aqueduct or the 4th ventricle).
- the obstruction of the communications with the subarachnoid cisterns – Magendie foramen, Luschka foramens; or the blockage of the basal sub-arachnoid space secondary to the sub-arachnoid hemorrhage or of an inflammatory origin. [9,10,12,13]

Therefore, there is a rapid increase in the intracranial pressure, which exceeds the normal limit values of 20 mm Hg. The increased intracranial pressure reduces the auto-regulation of the cerebral circulation.

There are significant ICP differences between the cerebrospinal compartments, which leads to the occurrence of cerebral herniation phenomena.

Clinical Presentation

The symptoms of hydrocephalus vary according to the illness age, the hydrocephalus progression type and the individual characteristics. The evolution of the ICH syndrome is rapid, and, if the appropriate therapy is not applied, the decompensated intracranial hypertension may occur

The usual signs in infants and young children are as follows:

- increase in the cranium dimensions,
- swelling of the anterior fontanelle,

- somnolence,
- vomiting,
- irritability,

In older children and adults, the symptomatology includes:

- cephalea preceded by vomiting,
- diplopia,
- development delay,
- disorders of walking, coordination, sphincter disorders,
- psychic disorders: of personality, of memory, irritability, etc.

In the case of the acute hydrocephalus, there is an escalation of the previous symptoms, or they are rapidly installed from the beginning:

- cephalea,
- vomiting,
- walking and equilibrium disorders,
- visual disorders.

Hydrocephalus Diagnosis

It is based on the clinical data and the paraclinical explorations: echography in infants and young children, cerebral computer tomography, nuclear magnetic resonance and intracranial pressure monitoring.[14,15,16,17]

Treatment

The purpose of the treatment is to reestablish the balance between the production and the absorption of the cerebrospinal fluid and the removal or avoidance of the causes that lead to a blockage of the cerebrospinal fluid circulation.[21,22,25,28,30,31]

Depending on the etiology and pathogenic mechanism, the following treatment is applied:

- the medical treatment that may diminish the production of the cerebrospinal fluid – acetazolamide,
- the etiologic neurosurgical treatment of the compressive lesion,
- the neurosurgical treatment of the cerebrospinal fluid drainage:
- a ventricular-peritoneal shunt is set up,
- the endoscopic ventriculostomy is applied for the 3rd ventricle,
- repeated, lumbar draining punctures are used. [21,22,24,25]

Intracranial Hypertension Due to Resorption Disorders

Intracranial hypertension due to resorption disorders or of a meningeal cause is the intracranial pressure increase caused by the reduction in the cerebrospinal fluid resorption due to various causes, which directly affect the resorption mechanisms. [2,6,10,17]

The diminished resorption of the cerebrospinal fluid can be caused by disorders of the cerebrospinal fluid resorption due to disorders of the membrane transfer mechanisms in the venous drainage system or to lesions of the anatomic structures that secure this transfer. The comparison between the two forms of ICH by disorders of the cerebrospinal fluid dynamics is presented in table 4.

Table 4. Comparison between the two forms of ICH by disorders of the cerebrospinal fluid dynamics:

ICH by dynamics disorders of the cerebrospinal fluid obstruction of the cerebrospinal fluid flow disorders of resorbtion CSF (meningeal ICH)	
Known etiology: obstruction of the cerebrospinal fluid circulation	Known etiology: meningeal inflammation, etc.
Obstructive hydrocephalus with periventricular or generalized edema	Communicating hydrocephalus with periventricular or generalized edema
ICH by dynamics disorders of the cerebrospinal fluid obstruction of the cerebrospinal fluid flow disorders of resorbtion CSF (meningeal ICH)	
Known etiology: obstruction of the cerebrospinal fluid circulation	Known etiology: meningeal inflammation, etc.
Rapid ICP increase	Moderate ICP increase
Critical ICP value ≈ 20 mm Hg	Critical ICP value ≈ 20 mm Hg
ICP differences between the cerebrospinal compartments	no ICP differences between the cerebrospinal compartments
The increased ICP decreases the auto-regulation of the cerebral circulation	The inflammatory vasculitis may affect the auto-regulation of the cerebral circulation
Short action duration of the increased ICP	Varied duration of the pressure – time fluctuation
Complete evolution towards decompensated ICH	Etiology dependent evolution, usually towards a complete or incomplete ICH syndrome
Neurosurgical treatment: etiologic or ventricular drainage	Symptomatic and/or etiologic treatment; sometimes a ventricular drainage in acute hydrocephalus

The pressure gradient changes from the drainage venous system by the venous sanguine pressure increase in the malformations of the Galien's vein (in children) or the longitudinal sinus thrombosis or the syndrome of the superior cavus vein, etc., reduce the cerebrospinal fluid resorption with the occurrence of the ICH syndrome, but the responsible pathogenic mechanism includes this form in the intracranial hypertension of vascular etiology.

The anatomic structures that ensure the drainage of the cerebrospinal fluid in the venous sinuses may be interested in acute meningitis, in sub-arachnoid hemorrhage of traumatisms, aneurisms, etc, in meningeal carcinomatosis, in chronic sarcoidosis meningitis, etc. Most frequently, there is a thickening of the leptomeninges by blocking Pachioni arachnoid corpuscles and by decreasing the absorption of the cerebrospinal fluid. The cerebrospinal fluid is accumulated in the ventricular system and a communicating hydrocephalus is produced, with a periventricular hydrocephalic brain edema and with a generally sub-acute intracranial hypertension syndrome, which is designated as the meningeal intracranial hypertension. [19,20,26,27,32]

The intracranial pressure increase is moderate and there are differences between the cerebrospinal compartments. Due to the meningeal inflammation, there may be an inflammatory vasculitis, which affects the superficial cerebral circulation in various degrees.

The clinical presentationand the type of intracranial pressure increase are similar to the intracranial hypertension syndrome in cases of obstructed circulation of the cerebrospinal fluid. The evolution depends on etiology, and it is usually headed towards a complete or incomplete ICH syndrome, usually with no occurrence of decompensation phenomena.

The treatment is symptomatic and/or etiologic depending on identifying etiology and ~~of~~ the pathogenic mechanisms; a ventricular drainage is rarely needed in order to prevent an acute hydrocephalus [21,23,26,29]

References

[1] Adamson DC, Dimitrov DF, Bronec PR. Upward transtentorial herniation, hydrocephalus, and cerebellar edema in hypertensive encephalopathy. *Neurologist.* 2005 11(3):171-5.

[2] Agrawal D, Chaturvedi DK. Shunt dependent hydrocephalus.*Br. J. Neurosurg.* 2004 ; 18(4):403

[3] Akbar M, Stippich C, Aschoff A. Magnetic resonance imaging and cerebrospinal fluid shunt valves. *N. Engl. J. Med.* 2005 29;353(13):1413-4

[4] Barbagallo GM, Platania N, Schonauer C. Long-term resolution of acute, obstructive, triventricular hydrocephalus by endoscopic removal of a third ventricular hematoma without third ventriculostomy. Case report and review of the literature. *J. Neurosurg.* 2005 ;102(5):930

[5] Bejjani GK. Association of the Adult Chiari Malformation and Idiopathic Intracranial Hypertension: more than a coincidence.*Med. Hypotheses.* 2003 ;60(6):859-63.

[6] Castano A, Volcy M, Garcia FA, Uribe CS,et al Headache in symptomatic intracranial hypertension secondary to leptospirosis: a case report. *Cephalalgia.* 2005 ;25(4):309-11.

[7] Cestari DM, Rizzo JF Intracranial hypertension following epidural blood patch. *Neurology.* 2003 . 11;61(9):1303.

[8] Czosnyka M, Czosnyka ZH, Richards HK, Pickard JD. Hydrodynamic properties of extraventricular drainage systems. *Neurosurgery.* 2003 ;52(3):619-23.

[9] Czosnyka ZH, Cieslicki K, Czosnyka M, Pickard JD. Hydrocephalus shunts and waves of intracranial pressure. *Med. Biol. Eng. Comput.* 2005 ;43(1):71-7.

[10] Eide PK. The relationship between intracranial pressure and size of cerebral ventricles assessed by computed tomography.*Acta Neurochir* (Wien). 2003 ;145(3):171-9;

[11] Forsyth R, Baxter P, Elliott T. Routine intracranial pressure monitoring in acute coma.*Cochrane Database Syst Rev.* 2001;(3):CD002043.

[12] Fritsch MJ, Doerner L, Kienke S, Mehdorn HM. Hydrocephalus in children with posterior fossa tumors: role of endoscopic third ventriculostomy. *J. Neurosurg.* 2005 ;103(1 Suppl):40-2

[13] Hamlat A, Heckly A, Doumbouya N, et al Epidural hematoma as a complication of endoscopic biopsy and shunt placement in a patient harboring a third ventricle tumor. *Pediatr. Neurosurg.* 2004 Sep-Oct; 40(5):245

[14] He XS, Zhang X. Giant calcified chronic subdural haematoma: a long term complication of shunted hydrocephalus.*J. Neurol. Neurosurg. Psychiatry.* 2005 ;76(3):367.

[15] Iannelli A, Rea G, Di Rocco C. CSF shunt removal in children with hydrocephalus.*Acta Neurochir (Wien).* 2005 ;147(5):503-7.

[16] Iencean St M Idiopathic intracranial hypertension and idiopathic normal pressure hydrocephalus: diseases with opposite pathogenesis? *Medical Hypotheses.* 2003 ;61(5-6):526-8.

[17] Iencean St M Pattern of increased intracranial pressure and classification of intracranial hypertension. *Journal of Medical Sciences*, 2004,.4,1 :52- 58

[18] Iencean St M Simultaneous hypersecretion of CSF and of brain interstitial fluid causes idiopathic intracranial hypertension. *Medical Hypotheses.* 2003 ;61(5-6):529-32.

[19] Joffe AR. Prognostic factors in adults with bacterial meningitis. *N. Engl. J. Med.* 2005, 3;352(5):512-5.

[20] Johnston M. The importance of lymphatics in cerebrospinal fluid transport.*Lymphat Res. Biol.* 2003;1(1):41-4.

[21] Kurtcuoglu V, Poulikakos D, Ventikos Y. Computational modeling of the mechanical behavior of the cerebrospinal fluid system. *J. Biomech. Eng.* 2005 ;127(2):264-9.

[22] Mathew P, Teasdale G, Bannan A, Oluoch-Olunya D. Neurosurgical management of cerebellar haematoma and infarct. *J. Neurol. Neurosurg. Psychiatry*. 1995; 59: 287–292.

[23] Olson S. The problematic slit ventricle syndrome. A review of the literature and proposed algorithm for treatment. *Pediatr. Neurosurg.* 2004 ;40(6):264-9.

[24] Perrin RG, Bernstein M. Tension pneumoventricle after placement of a ventriculoperitoneal shunt: a novel treatment strategy. Case report. *J. Neurosurg.* 2005 ;102(2):386-8.

[25] Psarros TG, Coimbra C. Endoscopic third ventriculostomy for patients with hydrocephalus and fourth ventricular cysticercosis: a review of five cases. *Minim. Invasive Neurosurg.* 2004 ; 47(6):346-9.

[26] Ramadan NM. Meningeal enhancement and low CSF pressure headache. An MRI study. *Cephalalgia.* 2005 ;25(7):558

[27] Riva M, Bacigaluppi S, Galli C, Citterio A, Collice M. Primary leptomeningeal gliomatosis: case report and review of the literature. *Neurol. Sci.* 2005 ;26(2):129-34.

[28] Rogg JM, Ahn SH, Tung GA, et al Prevalence of hydrocephalus in 157 patients with vestibular schwannoma. *Neuroradiology.* 2005 ;47(5):344-51.

[29] Singh D, Sachdev V, Singh AK, Sinha S. Endoscopic third ventriculostomy in post-tubercular meningitic hydrocephalus: a preliminary report.*Minim Invasive Neurosurg.* 2005 ;48(1):47-52.

[30] Sotelo J, Arriada N, Lopez MA. Ventriculoperitoneal shunt of continuous flow vs valvular shunt for treatment of hydrocephalus in adults.*Surg. Neurol.* 2005 ;63(3):197-203.

[31] van Toorn R, Georgallis P, Schoeman J. Acute cerebellitis complicated by hydrocephalus and impending cerebral herniation. *J. Child Neurol.* 2004 ;19(11):911-3.

[32] Wang KW, Chang WN, Chang HW, Wang HC, Lu CH. Clinical relevance of hydrocephalus in bacterial meningitis in adults.*Surg. Neurol.* 2005 ;64(1):61-5

[33] Woodworth GF, McGirt MJ, Williams MA, Rigamonti D. The use of ventriculoperitoneal shunts for uncontrollable intracranial hypertension without ventriculomegally secondary to HIV-associated cryptococcal meningitis. *Surg. Neurol.* 2005 ;63(6):529-31;

Chapter XIII

Idiopathic Intracranial Hypertension

General Data

Idiopathic intracranial hypertension is a syndrome characterized by the intracranial pressure increase in the absence of an expansive intracranial process, of hydrocephalus, of an intracranial infection, of dural venous sinus thrombosis, of hypertensive encephalopathy and without a neurotoxic etiology. The idiopathic intracranial hypertension partially corresponds to the old called "pseudotumor cerebri"; the term of benign intracranial hypertension has also been used, but it was subsequently dropped as it was noticed that the evolution of this illness can be accompanied by complications that exclude the idea of benignity (visual acuity decrease to cecity in some cases). [1,3,5,8]

This medical condition is described as a specific entity in Quincke's papers from 1893 and 1897 and then by Nonne in 1904, who is the first to use the term of pseudotumor cerebri. Various hypotheses are delivered in order to explain the causes and the pathogenic mechanisms of the illness.

The historic evolution of the knowledge on pseudotumor cerebri has been marked by several periods, which are characterized by the dominant pathogenic outlook and by the therapeutic orientation. Johnston identifies four periods in the historic development of the ideas on pseudotumor cerebri (2001):

- *the otologic stage* is dominated by the idea that the illness is associated to the infections of the middle ear, often extended to the dural sinuses, while the cause is the dynamic disorder of the cerebrospinal fluid. Symonds introduces the term of "otitic hydrocephalus" for this syndrome in the papers published in 1931- 1937, he suggests as a pathogenic mechanism the excessive secretion of cerebrospinal fluid at the level of the choroid plexuses or the decreased absorption of the cerebrospinal fluid through the arachnoid villi, recommending lumbar drainage as a treatment.
- *the neurosurgical stage* is dominated by the neuro-radiological explorations (ventriculography, pneumo-encephalography and angiography) and by debates on the intracranial compartments that are involved in ICH. There is an attempt in applying the neurosurgical therapy by lumbar punctures in moderate cases or by sub-

temporal decompression in refractory cases. Dandy (1937) suggests possible pathogenic mechanisms using the phrase “intracranial pressure without cerebral tumor” for the cases with a normal ventriculography and where the sub-temporal decompression has been used.

In 1955, Foley uses the term “benign intracranial hypertension”, which is to be used for several decades, and he defines this syndrome as follows: “prolonged intracranial hypertension without ventricular modifications, without focal neurological signs, without consciousness or intellectual disorders, the most important symptoms being a moderate cephalea, blurred sight, diplopia and sometimes tinnitus. The only signs are the papillary edema and the abducens paralysis. The cerebrospinal fluid has a normal composition. The prognosis is favorable, and the symptoms progressively diminish in several weeks or months.”

- *the neurological stage* has three important characteristics:

(a) the idea that the brain edema is the cause of the intracranial hypertension, which is based on the study of Sahs and Joynt from 1956,
(b) the introduction of diuretics and of steroids in the treatment of the brain edema,
(c) establishing the diagnosis using CT scan

The neurosurgical intervention is necessary only in cases that are refractory to the medical treatment.

- the neuro-ophthalmologic stage when the significance of visual disorders is reassessed (papillary edema, visual acuity decrease) in studies initiated by Corbett, 1982, returning to the decompression of the optic nerve in severe cases. The term of idiopathic intracranial hypertension is introduced by Buchheit and collaborators in 1969, gradually replacing the expression of benign intracranial hypertension, which Wall and George exclude in 1991 due to the visual complications, using only the term of idiopathic ICH. There are authors who use the term of “chronic intracranial hypertension” for idiopathic ICH although the chronic term may also be used in the case of a prolonged, compensated ICH, with a known etiology (intracranial sinus thrombosis, etc.)
- These stages are followed by the current period, which has brought about the differentiation between the forms of intracranial hypertension (based on the presented classification of intracranial hypertension) and the vascular intracranial hypertension is identified, after having been previously included in pseudotumor cerebri.
- the current stage:

- there are clear diagnosis criteria for the idiopathic intracranial hypertension and
- the comprehension of the illness pathogeny is based on the dynamics of the intracranial fluids, which allows the auto-regulation of the cerebral circulation within quasi-normal limits, despite the very high intracranial pressure. [2,3,4,6,7]

Diagnosis Criteria

According to Foley's classic definition, 1955, the idiopathic intracranial hypertension occurs as a diagnosis that may be established only by exclusion; moreover, even in Dandy's diagnosis criteria, modified by Wall, one of the diagnosis elements is the non-identification of another cause for the intracranial pressure increase. [2,9,10,12]

The diagnosis of idiopathic intracranial hypertension can be given only after the intracranial pressure has been measured and after a complete neuro-imagistic exploration.

The diagnosis criteria of the idiopathic intracranial hypertension, which are standardized by Friedman and Jacobson, and which are currently accepted are:

- the pressure of the cerebrospinal fluid is higher than 25 cm H_2O, that is higher than
- 18 - 20 mm Hg (by lumbar manometry performed after the CT or MRI exploration), the cerebrospinal fluid has a normal composition: normal or reduced cerebrospinal fluid proteins and normal cellularity,
- there are symptoms caused by the increased intracranial pressure: papillary edema, cephalea, with the absence of the neurological location signs (the abducens paresis is not a focal sign).
- the cerebral exploration using CT scan or MRI reveals normal cranial-cerebral aspects, a ventricular system with reduced dimensions may also be revealed (with a collapsed aspect) – without significance, or an empty sella; moreover, there is no clinical or neuro-imagistic suspicion of an intracranial venous sinus thrombosis.

In essence, these criteria limit the diagnosis of idiopathic intracranial hypertension to patients who have an increased cerebrospinal fluid pressure without a noticeable etiology.

Although it is not a diagnosis criteria, a guiding element is the predominance of the feminine sex, with a women / men proportion of approximately 2-8 / 1, with an interest in the age groups 20 - 50 years old, and with the maximum incidence in the third decade of age. [10,11,12, 13]

Various pathologic conditions can also be taken into account, when the idiopathic intracranial hypertension occurs more frequently: thus the global incidence of the idiopathic ICH is considered to be 1 - 2 cases / 100,000 but, in the case of young and obese women, it has been noticed that the incidence of idiopathic intracranial hypertension reaches 19-25 cases / 100,000.

In the case of a child with an idiopathic intracranial hypertension, there are several particularities compared to the adolescent and the adult, and, nowadays, certain diagnosis criteria have been proposed, which are slightly different from those for adults. In young children, gender and weight do not seem to be important factors. Pre-adolescents may manifest listlessness, irritability or somnolence, rather than headache; also dizziness and ataxia may occur. [12,14,15]

The proposed diagnostic criteria for pediatric idiopathic intracranial hypertension are as follows:

1. Prepubertal
2. Papilledema; symptoms or signs of generalized intracranial hypertension.
   Normal mental status.
3. Documented elevated intracranial pressure measured in the lateral decubitus position.
   Neonates: > 76 mm H20
   Age less than 8 with papilledema: > 180 mm H20
   Age 8 or above or less than 8 without papilledema: > 250 mm H20
4. Normal CSF composition (except in neonates)
5. Normal neuro-imaging studies are mandatory before diagnosing pediatric IIH:

   No evidence of hydrocephalus, mass, structural, or vascular lesion on MRI, with and without contrast, and MR venography (venous sinus thrombosis must also be excluded).
   Narrowing of the transverse sinuses is allowed.
6. Cranial nerve palsies are allowed if they are of no other identifiable etiology and if they improve with a reduction in the cerebrospinal fluid pressure or resolution of other signs and symptoms of intracranial hypertension.
7. No other identified cause of intracranial hypertension.

Etiology

The idiopathic intracranial hypertension is defined by the clinical existence of the intracranial hypertension syndrome, with very high ICP values and with a papillary edema in uncertain etiological conditions and due to pathogenic mechanisms that are difficult to establish. The term “associated factors” is used for the very diverse situations when the idiopathic intracranial hypertension occurs, without an etiopathogenic relationship. [15,16,17,18,19]

The pathological conditions where the idiopathic intracranial hypertension occurs are numerous and hard to systemize:

- metabolic and endocrine disorders:

  - if the global incidence of intracranial hypertension is estimated at 1 - 2/100,000, in young and obese women the incidence of idiopathic intracranial hypertension reaches 19 - 25/100,000. In the case of patients with idiopathic ICH, obesity is noted in a proportion of 80 - 90 % in women, in more than half of men, and in approximately one third of the children manifesting this syndrome.
  - hypothyroidism, parathyroid anomalies,
  - children treated with growth hormone,
  - the Addison illness.
- hypovitaminosis A;
- anemia due to Fe deficiency;
- system illnesses – lupus eritematos;

- medicines: - nalidixic acid, tetracycline, vitamin A, lithium carbonate, etc.,
- family syndromes, etc.

In numerous cases, a possible association can be determined with various conditions that are pathogenically suggestive, with not etiological notification; but there are plenty of cases when no etio-pathogenic relation can be revealed. [17,18]

Pathogenesis

The theories that have tried to explain the pathogeny of the idiopathic intracranial hypertension started from the identification of a very high increase in the intracranial pressure, in the absence of a space replacing lesion. According to Monro-Kellie theory regarding the limited volume of the intracranial content, the cause has been thought to be the increase in the volume of the endocranial fluids, based on a disorder of the secretion or absorption of the cerebrospinal fluid.

The increased resistance to the resorption of the cerebrospinal fluid with a diminished [17,19]resorption is one of the hypotheses on the pathogeny of the idiopathic intracranial hypertension. The relationship that governs the resorption of the cerebrospinal fluid is known (see Resorption of the Cerebrospinal Fluid):

CSF resorption rate = Pressure gradient (CSF – Venous sinus) / Flow resistance,

and, because the secretion of the cerebrospinal fluid is equal to its resorption in normal conditions, one may also write:

CSF production = Pressure gradient (CSF – Venous sinus) / Flow resistance,

which leads to:

CSF pressure = CSF production x Flow resistance + Venous pressure in the sagittal sinus

The diminished resorption of the cerebrospinal fluid means a slower circulation with the stagnation of the cerebrospinal fluid, which causes changes in its chemical composition, ; but one of the diagnosis criteria for the idiopathic ICH is that the cerebrospinal fluid has a normal composition: normal or reduced cerebrospinal fluid proteins and normal cellularity.

The increase in the venous pressure at the level of the sagittal sinus leads to the increase in the intracranial pressure, but the etiopathogeny is vascular and the syndrome is included in the vascular intracranial hypertension. [17,19,20,21]

The increase in the cerebrospinal fluid creation remains a possible pathogenic mechanism, but there is no hydrocephalus in the idiopathic intracranial hypertension; on the contrary, there may be a decrease in the ventricular dimensions.

The pathogeny of the idiopathic intracranial hypertension must be understood starting from the special characteristics of this syndrome and from the Monro-Kellie theory on the limited endocranial volume and on the mutual exchanges between the intracranial compartments. The characteristic features of the idiopathic intracranial hypertension syndrome reveal the functional and structural modifications that are possible due to the pathogenic mechanisms involved, as follows:

a. the ventricular system has small dimensions, which shows that there is no expansion towards the nervous parenchyma, therefore the parenchymatous pressure is equal to the intra-ventricular pressure from the beginning. This means that the parenchymatous pressure is in a balance with the increased pressure of the cerebrospinal fluid from the beginning, which is possible in two situations:

    - the pressure increase in the two compartments is simultaneous
    - the pressure increase happens first in the nervous parenchyma and then in the ventricular system

b. despite the very high values of the intracranial pressure, no cerebral hernias occur in the idiopathic intracranial hypertension, especially a hernia of cerebellar amygdales. In cases of increased intracranial pressure, the lumbar puncture is not recommended, but, in idiopathic intracranial hypertension, the lumbar puncture or the lumbar-peritoneal drainage improves the symptomatology and no cerebellar amygdale hernia occurs. The cerebral compliance is low in idiopathic ICH, which means that there is a small increase in the cerebral volume for a very high pressure increase, and this proves the pressure uniformity between the cerebral parenchyma and the ventricular system.
c. most frequently, the evolution registers a spontaneous improvement, despite the papillary edema and the possible visual deficits (which persist), which proves a minimal cerebral impact although the intracranial pressure has had very high values for long intervals.
d. there are rare cases of idiopathic intracranial hypertension with a unilateral papillary edema. The normal neuro-imagistic exploration and the measuring of the cerebrospinal fluid pressure have confirmed the diagnosis in these cases. The visual deficits and the evolution have been the same as in the case of patients with idiopathic ICH and a bilateral papillary edema. This suggests the fact that there are cases of idiopathic intracranial hypertension when the increased intracranial pressure does not generate a papillary edema by the non-transmission of increased pressure first of all towards the optical nerve.
e. the are acknowledged cases of idiopathic intracranial hypertension (with all the diagnosis criteria present) without the histological underlining of the brain edema. These characteristics show that the cerebral lesions are minimal, a possible condition only if the auto-regulation of the cerebral circulation is maintained active despite the very high values of the intracranial pressure. [21,22,24] Moreover, the image of the ventricular system with reduced dimensions despite the very high pressure of the

cerebrospinal fluid shows that the pressure of the surrounding cerebral parenchyma is discretely higher, indicating a trans-ependyma passage of the parenchymatous interstitial fluid towards ventricles.

f. the presence of tinnitus as intracranial pulsatile noises in more than 60 % of the patients with idiopathic intracranial hypertension can have the significance of a rapid and turbulent returning venous circulation. The reduced tinnitus at the jugular ipsilateral compression confirms the relation between the returning venous circulation and the presence of these intracranial pulsatile noises. The reduced tinnitus after the decompressive lumbar puncture also shows that the decreased quantity of cerebrospinal fluid reduces the venous drainage.

A hypothesis has been launched according to which the tinnitus, together with the vertigo and the nausea, are secondary to the compression of the acoustic-vestibular nerve caused by the increase in the intracranial pressure. [18,23,25,26]

The fact that these symptoms diminish after the lumbar puncture, which decreases the ICP, would support this hypothesis, but the fact that the tinnitus is also reduced by jugular ipsilateral compression supports the relationship with the returning venous circulation.

All these aspects prove that the existence of an increased quantity of cerebrospinal fluid in idiopathic intracranial hypertension is followed by a rapid fluid circulation and resorption.

The pathogenic mechanisms are based on the dynamics of the intracranial fluids, and they correspond to the circuit of the fluids that justify the increased pressure of the cerebrospinal fluid and allow the maintenance of the cerebral circulatory auto-regulation with a normal nervous functioning. [26,27,28,29]

The dynamics of the intracranial fluids in the case of the idiopathic intracranial hypertension can include several fluid circuits that concord to the brain edema and to the increased parenchymatous pressure, which is equal to the increased pressure of the cerebrospinal fluid, concomitantly to the maintenance of the cerebral sanguine circulation, which may explain the good clinical condition:

1. hyper-production of interstitial fluid with increased resorption at the level of the brain blood barrier – which explains the increased parenchymatous pressure and the hyper-production of cerebrospinal fluid, which may explain the increased pressure of the cerebrospinal fluid, with increased resorption at the level of the venous sinuses, as well as intense and rapid exchanges from the interstitial fluid towards the cerebrospinal fluid at the level of the ventricular wall, trans-ependyma, and at the trans-cerebral pial level, which explains the pressure equilibrium between the cerebral parenchyma – ventricles, with a rapid venous drainage;
2. hyper-production of cerebrospinal fluid, increased resorption at the level of venous sinuses with rapid venous drainage;
3. hyper-production of interstitial fluid by modification of the brain-blood barrier, normal production of cerebrospinal fluid, but with increased exchanges from the interstitial fluid towards the trans-ependyma cerebrospinal fluid and at the trans-cerebral pial level, with a rapid venous drainage.

The increased production of cerebrospinal fluid at the level of the choroid plexuses, and then with increased resorption, cannot explain the brain edema and the pressure equilibrium at the level of the nervous parenchyma – ventricular system.

The brain edema occurs due to the impact on the brain-blood barrier, generating an increased flux of interstitial fluid, with an increase in the intra-parenchymatous pressure.

The maintenance of the cerebral sanguine circulation within normal limits imposes the decrease in the parenchymatous pressure, which can be achieved through an increased resorption of the interstitial fluid and / or by the trans-ependyma passage in ventricles, and a trans-pial passage in the sub-arachnoid space. The resulting increased quantity of cerebrospinal fluid does not cause a ventricular dilatation because an increased resorption occurs; the ventricular system is usually reduced in volume, which suggests the fact that the trans-ependyma fluid circuit is predominant for the increase in the volume of cerebrospinal fluid, compared to the production at the level of the choroid plexuses. [17,19,29,30]

The increased resorption of the cerebrospinal fluid corresponds quantitatively to the trans-ependyma exchange from the volume increased interstitial fluid, ensuring the intracranial circuit of fluids.

The dynamics of the relations intracranial pressure – intracranial volume is expressed by the circulation of fluids, which allows the existence of an increased fluid pressure, although this pressure does not act significantly on the endocranial structures and on the cerebral circulation, which is maintained within normal limits.

The most probable pathogenic mechanism is the impacts on the brain blood barrier of the hyper-production of interstitial fluid and an extracellular brain edema; the cerebrospinal fluid is produced normally; there are increased exchanges from the interstitial fluid towards the cerebrospinal fluid at the trans-ependyma level and at the trans-cerebral pial level; an increased resorption of the cerebrospinal fluid is produced, and there is a rapid venous efflux.

The clinical sign of the rapid and possibly turbulent venous flow is the synchronic tingles with a pulse, which are frequent in idiopathic intracranial hypertension.

One may consider that an uncertain cause generates impacts on the brain blood barrier with the gradual appearance of the brain edema due to the increase in the interstitial fluid.

The trans-ependyma exchange between the interstitial fluid of the edema from the cerebral parenchyma towards the cerebrospinal fluid, by means of which pressure is equalized, is followed by the increased resorption of the cerebrospinal fluid, maintaining the cerebral circulation, and representing a compensating mechanism. This mechanism is efficient and it allows the cerebral circulatory auto-regulation when there is a progressive injury of the brain-blood barrier, the interstitial fluid volume increases slowly and the brain edema is also gradually installed. [12,17,18,31,32]

The trans-ependymal and trans-pial circuit of the interstitial fluid towards the cerebrospinal fluid is the fundamental element for this compensating mechanism of pressure increase.

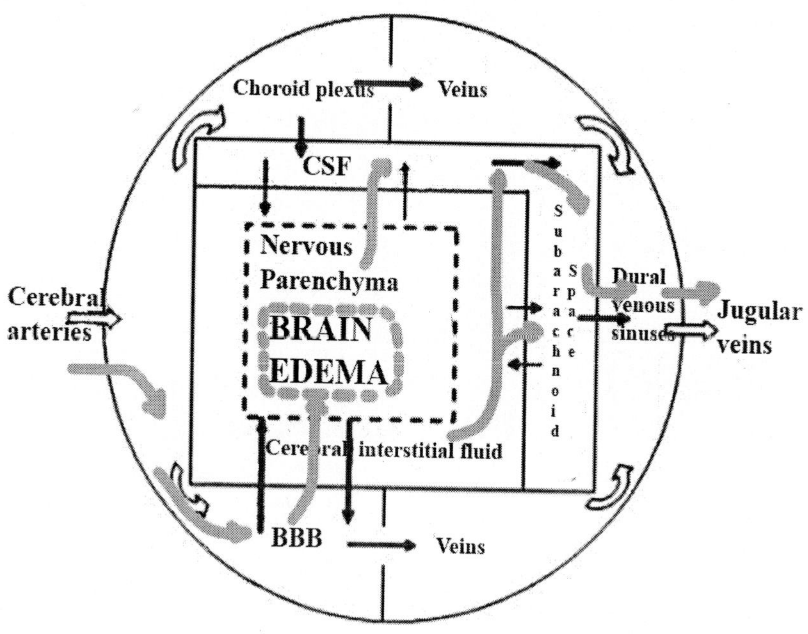

Figure 58. Hydrodynamic model of pathogeny in idiopathic intracranial hypertension

The increase in the intracranial pressure is extremely slow, with a chronic aspect. This very slow increase in the intracranial pressure allows good pressure compensation and an almost normal maintenance of the cerebral sanguine flux. The pathogenic ICP values are very high, of up to 60 - 80 mm Hg, values that may be maintained on a plateau for long periods.[31,32,36,35]

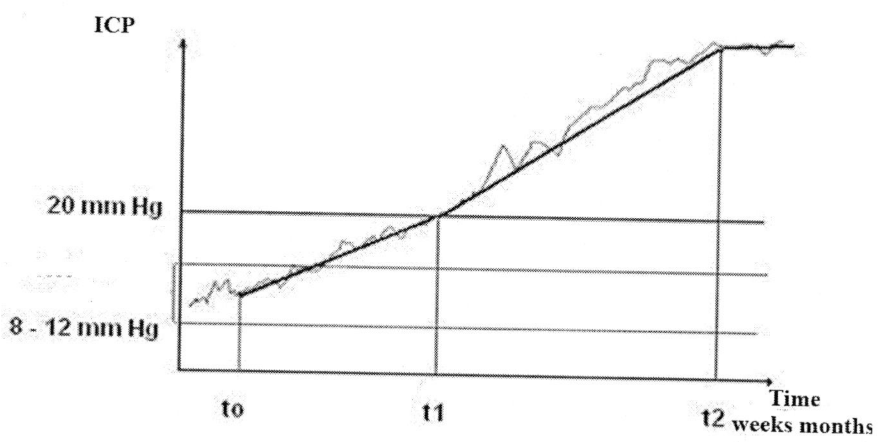

Figure 59. ICP increase in idiopathic ICH, with prolonged infraclinical period and with an extremely long duration of pathological pressure values.

This pathogenic mechanism, which is based on the compensation of the fluid pressure increase by means of a gradual accentuation of the trans-ependymal circuit functioning and the trans-pial transfer of the interstitial fluid towards the cerebrospinal fluid, explains:

- the absence of hydrocephalus despite the increased pressure of the cerebrospinal fluid, through increased fluid resorption,
- the small dimensions of the ventricular system due to the initially increased pressure at the level of the nervous parenchyma, and subsequently balanced by the transfer of the interstitial fluid towards the cerebrospinal fluid,
- the good clinical condition due to the auto-regulation of the cerebral circulation, because the increased intracranial pressure has a reduced action on the endocranial structures in the dynamic conditions of the rapid fluid circuit;
- the brain edema frequently exists due to the dysfunction of the brain blood barrier and to the existence of an increased quantity of interstitial fluid; at the same time, in some cases, the brain edema may be reduced or even absent because the fluid transfer towards the cerebrospinal fluid is sufficiently rapid and intense for the brain edema not to be significant.

Clinical Presentation

The clinical syndrome generally includes only cephalea; sometimes visual disorders and oculomotor pareses occur gradually (visual acuity decrease).

Cephalea is present in most cases of idiopathic intracranial hypertension. Cephalea is diffuse and it can seldom be localized. It is frequently continuous, but of a reduced or moderate, bearable intensity, sometimes with irregular exacerbations, with a pulsatile aspect and with a feeling of a cephalic burden. It may be more intense in the morning, depending on the nocturnal increase in the intracranial pressure, although this is not a characteristic of the idiopathic intracranial hypertension. Generally, it is not accompanied by vomiting, and the usual antalgics are efficient. [13,14,32,33]

The idiopathic ICH cephalea has a slow, gradual character, it may reach moderate exacerbations and it maintains its characteristics for long periods.

Cephalea is installed later than the occurrence and outlining of the papillary edema.

There is no connection between cephalea and the values of the intracranial pressure, since there are very high increases in the intracranial pressure (with important impacts on the eye fundus) without cephalea or with a bearable cephalea.

The temporary loss of sight frequently occurs in patients with idiopathic intracranial hypertension, which are thought to evoke the idiopathic ICH syndrome. The phenomenon consists of a sudden cecity of a few seconds, usually 5 seconds or less, but always lasting for less than half a minute, followed by the recovery of sight. The frequency of these visual eclipses is not correlated to the aspect of the papillary edema, and no clear correlation can be established with a possible evolution towards the visual acuity decrease.

The visual acuity can decrease, usually at later stages, and in up to 10 – 15 % of cases, there is a significant decrease in the visual acuity, sometimes to cecity. The visual acuity decrease occurs gradually, or the cecity can appear, in less than a day. The reduced visual acuity is untreatable, and this sequel has excluded the term of benign intracranial hypertension.

The tinnitus are present in more than half of the patients with idiopathic intracranial hypertension, they are frequently pulsatile and unilateral, and sometimes they are associated to a hearing decrease. The ipsilateral jugular compression or the lumbar drainage of the cerebrospinal fluid diminishes the tingles.

The external oculomotor nerve paresis may be unilateral or bilateral, and it may cause a horizontal diplopia. The abducens paresis is not considered to be a neurological location sign as it is secondary to the intracranial pressure increase caused by various etiologies.

The presence of hyposmia has been recently described in some patients with idiopathic ICH, and a hypothesis has been launched according to which the intracranial pressure increase compromises the olphactive fibers, similar to the impacts on the optic nerve in ICH.

As the CSF drainage is also achieved using the important contribution of the of the olfactory perineural sheath, the olphactive assessment could be a diagnosis element for the idiopathic intracranial hypertension when hyposmia is acknowledged to be a constant component of the clinical presentation. [6,7,9,17]

In case of children with idiopathic ICH, symptoms vary from a complete clinical presentationwith cephalea, sight disorders, affectivity disorders and cranial nerve pareses, to the absence of any symptom, in the case of an asymptomatic idiopathic intracranial hypertension, with a occasional discovery of the papillary edema.

Paraclinical Explorations

1. Ophthalmologic exploration

The eye fundus examination reveals the papillary edema, which is present in all cases of idiopathic intracranial hypertension; it has a long development, with a gradual installation, and there is a frequent relationship with the decrease in the visual acuity. Sometimes, the progression of the papillary edema towards atrophy may not be stopped. The papillary edema occurs gradually a few weeks after the intracranial pressure begins to increase, passing through the stages of papillary contour blurring, erasure of the papillary contour, manifest papillary edema with venous stasis and pericapillary hemorrhages. The evolution is long and the papillary edema can be unequal in the two eyes. Usually, the idiopathic intracranial hypertension presents a discordance between cephalea, which is present but minor, and the severe papillary edema, which can lead to the visual acuity decrease. The papillary edema decreases slowly, for up to half a year, after the other symptoms have disappeared.

The repeated ophthalmologic examination is compulsory in order to reveal the reduced visual acuity in good time, as it can occur in cases of idiopathic intracranial hypertension with a long development. [16,17,35]

There may be changes in the visual field that are not characteristics because they are similar to those induced by the papillary edema generated by other causes.

2. The neuro-imagistic cerebral exploration using computer tomography reveals normal cranial-cerebral aspects, while later it can be seen that the ventricular system has reduced dimensions or the image of an empty sella. The exploration of the cerebral circulation by

catheter angiography – venous time, angio-CT or MRI venography – excludes a thrombosis of intracranial venous sinus.

3. The exploration of the cerebrospinal fluid can be performed by lumbar puncture after the neuro-imagistic exploration that has excluded an expansive intracranial process. The assessment of the fluid pressure by lumbar manometry is compulsory, and it represents a diagnosis criterion for the idiopathic ICH.

The CSF pressure is higher than 25 cm H_2O, which means higher than 18 - 20 mm Hg.

The cerebrospinal fluid has a normal composition from a biochemical point of view and a normal cellularity. [14,17,21]

Differential Diagnosis

The differential diagnosis is applied at first for the clinical symptomatology, i.e. it is the differential diagnosis of a prolonged cephalea, which requires the performance of a paraclinical exploration, first of all the performance of an eye fundus examination and then the neuro-imagistic cerebral exploration. Some patients require an ORL consultation for tingles. The idiopathic intracranial hypertension diagnosis is practically a diagnosis that excludes the other causes that can bring about the intracranial pressure increase.

Evolution

The evolution of the idiopathic intracranial hypertension is generally remissive, often spontaneous, but there can be up to 10% cases of relapse.

An aspect that is considered to evoke idiopathic ICH is the discordance between the patient's apparently good or satisfactory condition and the actual evolution of the intracranial hypertension with very increased ICP values and the presence of the papillary edema. In 10–15 % of the cases with a long evolution, and which are usually not monitored, a diminished visual acuity may occur, sometimes to cecity. The decrease in the visual acuity is final, and the terminology of benign intracranial hypertension is no longer used due to the occurrence of this sequel.

The clinical evolution is towards an incomplete syndrome of intracranial hypertension without decompensation.

Treatment

In the case of a benign intracranial hypertension diagnosis, a therapy is used depending on the possible associated factors – metabolic and hormonal corrections, exclusion of certain medication, etc.

A symptomatic treatment is applied for cephalea, and cerebral anti-edematous substances are administered, such as dexamethasone, or diuretics (acetazolamide, furosemide) in order to decrease the intracranial pressure. [1,17,22]

In some cases of obese patients, the weight loss is followed by an obvious clinical improvement, and by the progressive reduction of the papillary edema.

Moreover, repeated lumbar punctures and lumbar-peritoneal shunting have been used with good clinical results. An approximate quantity of 30 ml CSF is evacuated by lumbar puncture or the cerebrospinal fluid is drained until the intracranial pressure, which is measured by the lumbar method, is seen to have decreased to approximately half of the initial value.

The lumbar-peritoneal shunting drains the excessive CSF and the symptomatology disappears within less than a month; the shunting revising rate may reach to 50 %.

In some cases of significant visual acuity decrease, there has been an attempt to decompress the optic nerve by performing fenestrations at the level of the optic nerve sheath in order to produce a decrease of the papillary edema, but the results are not always favorable.

References

[1] Adelson PD, Bratton SL, Carney NA, Chesnut RM, et al Threshold for treatment of intracranial hypertension. *Pediatr. Crit Care Med.* 2003 ;4(3 Suppl):S25-7.

[2] Adelson PD, Bratton SL, Carney NA, Chesnut RM,et al Intracranial pressure monitoring technology. Pediatr Crit Care Med. 2003 ;4(3 Suppl):S28-30.

[3] Bari L, Choksi R, Roach ES. Otitic hydrocephalus revisited. *Arch. Neurol.* 2005 ;62(5): 824 -5

[4] Bejjani GK. Association of the Adult Chiari Malformation and Idiopathic Intracranial Hypertension: more than a coincidence.*Med. Hypotheses.* 2003 ;60(6):859-63.

[5] Chamberlain CE, Fitzgibbon E, Wassermann EM, et al Idiopathic intracranial hypertension following kidney transplantation: A case report and review of the literature. *Pediatr. Transplant.* 2005 ; 9 (4):545-50.

[6] Digre KB. Idiopathic intracranial hypertension headache.*Curr. Pain Headache Rep.* 2002 ; 6(3):217-25.

[7] Digre KB. Not so benign intracranial hypertension.*BMJ.* 2003 22;326(7390):613-4.

[8] Drake J. Slit-ventricle syndrome. *J. Neurosurg.* 2005 ;102(3 Suppl):257-8.

[9] Duggal HS. Idiopathic intracranial hypertension presenting with psychiatric symptoms. *J. Neuropsychiatry Clin. Neurosci.* 2005 ;17(3):426-7

[10] Farb RI, Vanek I, Scott JN, Mikulis DJ, Willinsky RA,et al Idiopathic intracranial hypertension: the prevalence and morphology of sinovenous stenosis. *Neurology.* 2003 13;60(9):1418-24.

[11] Francis PJ, Haywood S, Rigden S, Calver DM, Clark G. Benign intracranial hypertension in children following renal transplantation. *Pediatr. Nephrol.*2003; 18(12):1265-9.

[12] Friedman DI. Medication-induced intracranial hypertension in dermatology. Am J Clin Dermatol. 2005;6(1):29-37.

[13] Giuseffi V, Wall M, Siegel PZ, Rojas PB. Symptoms and disease associations in idiopathic intracranial hypertension: a case-control study. *Neurology* 1991; 41:239-244.

[14] Gjerris, F., Sarensen, P. S., Vorstrup, S., et al.: Intracranial pressure, conductance to cerebrospinal fluid outflow, and cerebral blood flow in patients with benign intracranial hypertension (pseudotumor cerebri). *Ann. Neurol.* 1985, 17:158,.

[15] Huna-Baron R, Kupersmith MJ. Idiopathic intracranial hypertension in pregnancy. *J. Neurol.* 2002 ;249(8):1078-81.

[16] Hung HL, Kao LY, Huang CC. Ophthalmic features of idiopathic intracranial hypertension. *Eye.* 2003 ;17(6):793-5.

[17] Iencean St M Idiopathic intracranial hypertension and idiopathic normal pressure hydrocephalus: diseases with opposite pathogenesis? *Medical Hypotheses.* 2003 ;61(5-6):526-8.

[18] Iencean St M Pattern of increased intracranial pressure and classification of intracranial hypertension. *Journal of Medical Sciences,* 2004,.4,.1 :52- 58

[19] Iencean St M Simultaneous hypersecretion of CSF and of brain interstitial fluid causes idiopathic intracranial hypertension. *Medical Hypotheses.* 2003 ;61(5-6):529-32.

[20] Jacob S, Rajabally YA. Intracranial hypertension induced by rofecoxib.*Headache.* 2005; 45(1):75-6.

[21] King JO, Mitchell PJ, Thomson KR, et al: Cerebral venography and manometry in idiopathic intracranial hypertension. *Neurology,*1995, 45:2224–2228,

[22] Lee AG, Pless M, Falardeau J,et al The use of acetazolamide in idiopathic intracranial hypertension during pregnancy. *Am. J. Ophthalmol.* 2005 ;139(5):855-9.

[23] Lochhead J, Elston JS. Doxycycline induced intracranial hypertension.*BMJ.* 2003 22; 326(7390):641-2.

[24] Najjar MW, Azzam NI, Khalifa MA. Pseudotumor cerebri: disordered cerebrospinal fluid hydrodynamics with extra-axial CSF collections. *Pediatr. Neurosurg.*2005; 41(4):212-5.

[25] Ng YT, Bodensteiner JB. Idiopathic intracranial hypertension in the pediatric population. *J. Child Neurol.* 2003 , 18(6):440 .

[26] Owler BK, Parker G, Halmagyi GM, Pseudotumor cerebri syndrome: venous sinus obstruction and its treatment with stent placement. J Neurosurg. 2003 ;98(5):1045-55.

[27] Rickels MR, Nichols CW. Pseudotumor cerebri in patients with Cushing's disease. *Endocr. Pract.* 2004;10(6):492-6.

[28] Serratrice J, Granel B, Conrath J,et al Benign intracranial hypertension and thyreostimulin suppression hormonotherapy.Am J Ophthalmol. 2002 ;134(6):910-1.

[29] Sismanis, A., Butts, F. M., and Hughes, G. B.: Objective tinnitus in benign intracranial hypertension: An update. *Laryngoscope,*1990, 100:33,

[30] Stanley TV. Idiopathic intracranial hypertension presenting as hemiplegic migraine. *Acta Paediatr.* 2002;91(8):980-2.

[31] Tabassi A, Salmasi AH, Jalali M. Serum and CSF vitamin A concentrations in idiopathic intracranial hypertension. *Neurology.* 2005 14;64(11):1893-6.

[32] Vorstman EB, Niemann DB, Molyneux AJ, Pike MG. Benign intracranial hypertension associated with arteriovenous malformation. *Dev. Med Child Neurol.* 2002 ;44(2):133-5.

[33] Weber KT, Singh KD, Hey JC. Idiopathic intracranial hypertension with primary aldosteronism: report of 2 cases.*Am. J. Med Sci.* 2002 ;324(1):45-50..

[34] Weig SG. Asymptomatic idiopathic intracranial hypertension in young children. *J. Child Neurol.* 2002 ;17(3):239-41.

[35] Wraige E, Chandler C, Pohl KR. Idiopathic intracranial hypertension: is papilloedema inevitable? *Arch. Dis. Child.* 2002 ;87(3):223-4.

Chapter XIV

Evolution and Prognosis

The evolution of the intracranial hypertension depends on the etiology, on the early diagnosis and on the immediate commencement of an appropriate treatment.

From an etiopathogenic point of view, there are three stages of the intracranial hypertension depending on the values of the intracranial pressure:

- the initial stage when the intracranial pressure increases above the usual values of 15 – 16 mm Hg, but is below 20 mm Hg, which is a stage that is not accompanied by any clinical signs,
- the stage when the intracranial stage exceeds the normal threshold value of 20 mm Hg, and the clinical signs of the intracranial hypertension syndrome appear. The clinical start depends on the efficiency of the compensating mechanisms of the ICP increase.
- the decompensation stage, caused by surpassing ~~of~~ the compensating mechanisms of the intracranial pressure increase, and having a characteristic clinical presentation. {1,2,3,4]

These stages have a clinical correspondent that is manifested through specific clinical symptoms caused by the changes in the volume – intracranial pressure relation and by the compensating capacity of the ICP increase.

The initial ICP increase up to the normal limit value is a signal of alarm from a pressure point of view, but it does not present a clinical symptomatology. Once the normal ICP value is exceeded, clinical signs of intracranial hypertension appear; therefore the ICH clinical presentation can only be correlated to pressure values of more than 20 mm Hg.

As far as the efficiency of the pressure increase compensating mechanisms is concerned, the clinical presentationof the intracranial hypertension can be described as:

- the starting period of the ICH syndrome,
- the complete ICH syndrome,
- the decompensation of the intracranial hypertension,
- the remission period of the ICH syndrome,

- the late sequelae period.

These clinical stages can be consecutive in the development of the untreated intracranial hypertension or the development can stop at a clinical stage depending on the etiopathogeny of the illness or on the treatment applied. The development towards decompensation is stopped or the remission of the intracranial hypertension syndrome is possible by applying an appropriate treatment as soon as possible. If an efficient treatment is applied, stopping the ICH decompensation, and the evolution of the illness is favorable, there can be persisting symptoms that represent sequels of an incomplete cerebral lesion, stopped in its development, such as the hydrocephalus produced by CSF dynamic disorders or the ophthalmologic disorders in idiopathic ICH. [3,4,5]

The starting and the status periods of the intracranial hypertension include the complete or partial classical chart of the ICH syndrome; the decompensation of the intracranial hypertension includes the worsening of the symptoms of the previous stage or their sudden installation with consciousness disorders or coma.

Depending on the starting method on the subsequent evolution, the intracranial hypertension can manifest itself as:

- an acute form, with the initial installation of the symptoms corresponding to decompensation;
- the sub-acute form, with a slowly progressive increase in the intracranial pressure up to the normal threshold value, after which the ICP increase may be rapid, and the decompensation occurs, as in the case of sub-dural chronic hematomas;
- a type with prolonged development, with a chronic aspect, in the endocranial lesions with a slow expansion, or in the forms of idiopathic ICH. The symptoms occur successively and they escalate gradually depending on the gradual exhaustion of the compensating means. In this case, a stage is reached when the compensating possibilities are exhausted and there is a severe clinical presentationas in the acute form.

The clinical presentationof the decompensated intracranial hypertension or the ICH illness is severe. The consequences of the intracranial hypertension occur due to the impact on the cerebral circulation and/or by the cerebral herniation, and they happen because of the ischemia, hemorrhage and the direct compression of the vital centers of the brainstem.

The remission period of the intracranial hypertension syndrome is characterized by the progressive reduction of the symptomatology, most often within a relatively short interval of time with a recovery from coma and a significant neurological improvement or a diminution of symptoms and the stop of the development towards decompensation.

Post-intracranial hypertension sequels are considered to be the symptoms or the syndromes that persist for a long period after the remission of an ICH syndrome: oculomotor pareses, comitial crises, psychic disorders, hydrocephalus that ~~ahs~~ has required a ventricular drainage, persistence of eye fundus modifications, visual acuity reduction etc. [4,5,6,7,8]

References

[1] Allan R, Chaseling R. Subtemporal decompression for slit-ventricle syndrome: successful outcome after dramatic change in intracranial pressure wave morphology. Report of two cases. *J. Neurosurg.* 2004 ;101(Suppl):214-7.

[2] Barbagallo GM, Platania N, Schonauer C. Long-term resolution of acute, obstructive, triventricular hydrocephalus by endoscopic removal of a third ventricular hematoma without third ventriculostomy. *J. Neurosurg.* 2005 ;102(5):930-4..

[3] Drake JM. The surgical management of pediatric hydrocephalus.*Neurosurgery.* 2008 ;62 Suppl 2:633-40

[4] Iencean St M Pattern of increased intracranial pressure and classification of intracranial hypertension. *Journal of Medical Sciences,* 2004,.4,.1 :52- 58

[5] Kang JK, Lee IW.Long-term follow-up of shunting therapy Childs Nerv Syst. 1999;15(11-12):711-7

[6] Oi S. Diagnosis, outcome, and management of fetal abnormalities: fetal hydrocephalus.*Childs Nerv Syst.* 2003 ;19(7-8):508-16.

[7] Piovesan EJ, Lange MC, Do Rocio Maia Piovesan L et al Long-term evolution of papilledema in idiopathic intracranial hypertension: Observations concerning two cases

[8] Arquivos de Neuro-Psiquiatria 2002, . 60, 2b, . 453-457

[9] Santamarta D, Martin-Vallejo J. Evolution of intracranial pressure during the immediate postoperative period after endoscopic third ventriculostomy.*Acta Neurochir Suppl.* 2005;95:213-7.

Chapter XV

Intracranial Hypertension Treatment

General Data

The treatment of intracranial hypertension depends on the type of intracranial hypertension and on the developmental stage of the illness. The treatment is first of all an etiologic one in order to remove the cause that has caused the intracranial pressure increase; simultaneously, there is an attempt to stop the pathogenic mechanisms that impact on the nervous structures, and a symptomatic treatment is applied in order to reduce the intensity of the clinical syndrome.

The term of etiologic treatment refers to the etiology of the intracranial hypertension, that is to the immediate cause that generates the intracranial pressure increase: for instance, in the case of a cerebral metastasis leading to ICH, the name of etiologic treatment is given to the action of metastasis extirpation, and it has no connection to the etiology and the therapy of the original neoplasia. [1,2,3,4,65,15]

The intracranial hypertension treatment can be complex by combining three therapeutic methods used concomitantly or successively, or only the pathogenic therapy and the symptomatic one are used, depending on the clinical stage and the paraclinical explorations.

The type of intracranial hypertension establishes the treatment that must be applied:

1. the treatment is etiologic in:

- expansive intracranial processes: cerebral tumors, intracranial hematomas, cerebral abscesses, hydatid cyst, etc., in the case of parenchymatous intracranial hypertension,
- hypertensive encephalopathy in the case of vascular intracranial hypertension,
- thrombosis of intracranial vessels, venous or arterial, in the case of vascular intracranial hypertension,
- CSF circulation disorders due to the existence of a ventricular or paraventricular tumor with the occurrence of an obstructive hydrocephalus,
- CSF resorption disorders in acute meningitis.
-

2. the pathogenic treatment is applied in:

- all the ICH cases with known etiology, which are mentioned above, in order to stop the development of the pathogenic mechanisms that have already started,
- the parenchymatous intracranial hypertension due to posttraumatic brain edema, hypoxic brain edema caused by secondary posttraumatic cerebral ischemia or in the case of sub-arachnoid hemorrhage, general intoxications with neurotoxins (endogenous or exogenous), etc.
- the vascular intracranial hypertension due to cerebral venous thrombosis, thrombosis of superior sagittal sinus with a decrease in the venous drainage and the blockage of the CSF absorption, or in the case of the secondary ischemic brain edema in the ischemic stroke caused by the occlusion or the stenosis of the great cerebral vessels,
- intracranial hypertension due to CSF dynamic disorder
- idiopathic intracranial hypertension especially in order to block the development of certain complications depending on possible pathogenic mechanisms.

3. symptomatic treatment:

- all the cases of intracranial hypertension, when the etiologic and/or pathogenic therapy is applied, benefit from the symptomatic treatment, depending on the presented symptomatology,
- in idiopathic intracranial hypertension. [1,215,27,28,46]

Based on the manifested clinical syndrome, there may be several situations that correspond to the evolutionary stages of intracranial hypertension:

- the patient is conscious and the cerebral exploration reveals a lesion that may cause the development of an intracranial hypertension syndrome – the treatment is etiologic and it addresses the lesion that may cause ICH,
- the patient is conscious with incipient ICH signs, therefore with a compensated ICH syndrome, with or without focal neurological signs – the treatment is etiologic, pathogenic and symptomatic,
- the patient is in a critical condition, with consciousness disorders, with a decompensating ICH syndrome or in a coma due to the decompensation of the intracranial hypertension – the treatment is etiologic, pathogenic and symptomatic, and it is applied immediately.

Therapeutic Recommendations

Etiologic Treatment

I. If there is an expansive intracranial process that caused the intracranial hypertension syndrome, the etiologic treatment consists in the surgical intervention for the lesion removal.

In numerous situations, the neurosurgical techniques allow the ablation of that particular expansive intracranial process:

- the extirpation of the cerebral tumors is complete or partial, depending on the tumor location relative to the eloquent nervous structures, and depending on the benign or malign character of the neoformation. The removal of the neoformation makes The supplementary endocranial volume disappears as a first moment in the development of the intracranial hypertension, as well as removing the compressive effect on the CSF circulation paths and the edematous effect on the adjacent nervous parenchyma.
- the expansive traumatic lesions, with or without a traumatic brain edema, are surgically solved by the evacuation of the traumatic hematomas, the removal of the edematous cerebral dilaceration, etc.,
- other expansive intracranial lesions, non-tumor or non-traumatic lesions, such as the cerebral abscess, the dural empyema, the hydatid cyst, etc., are surgically solved, usually by a complete evacuation.[4,6,8]

II. In the case of hypertensive encephalopathy, the etiologic treatment is the treatment of the hypertensive crises with a gradual, but fast enough, return, to normal values of the blood pressure, concomitantly to the brain edema decrease and the clinical improvement of the ICH syndrome.

III. In the case of the vascular intracranial hypertension, due to cerebral venous thrombosis, thrombosis of superior sagittal sinus, etc., anti-thrombotic and anti-coagulant substances may be used.

IV. In the ischemic stroke caused by the occlusion or stenosis of the great vessels, substances with fibrinolytic action may be used: intravenous thrombolysis, fibrinogen degrading enzymes, etc. The thrombotic occlusion of the Sylvian artery can benefit from an extra-intracranial anastomosis with the superficial temporal artery. The carotid endarteroctomy and the angioplasty, with the mechanic removal of the sanguine coagulum or with the installation of an arterial stent, have been used in emergency cases, but certain procedures are presented especially as prophylactic surgical treatments for the cerebral stroke in patients with repeated transitory ischemic cerebral vascular accidents.

V. The intracranial hypertension, due to CSF resorption disorders, secondary to an acute meningitis benefits from the etiologic treatment of the bacterial meningitis, which decreases the meningeal inflammation and reduces the changes in CSF resorption.

VI. In intracranial hypertension of acute liver failure with endotoxic etiology, the etiologic treatment consists of performing a hepatic transplant. The decision on the performance of the hepatic transplant is made based on the neurological prognosis monitoring the intracranial pressure in the fulminating case of a hepatic failure of a degree ≥ 3, (West Haven Criteria of Altered Mental Status In Hepatic Encephalopathy).

VII. In the intracranial hypertension of the posterior reversible encephalopathy syndrome (PRES) with a non-hypertensive etiology, due to the neurotoxic action of certain immunosuppressors or cytostatics, the treatment is etiologic, and it consists of interrupting the causing medication, with the progressive improvement within a few days. [4,9,11,28]

Pathogenic Treatment

The pathogenic treatment is used in all types of intracranial hypertension in order to stop the pathogenic mechanisms by means of which various causes bring about the intracranial pressure increase, and which cause the compensating capacities of the endocranial pressure increases to be exceeded. [3,4,9,19,20,22]

The purpose of the pathogenic treatment is:

- to act on the development of the brain edema, and once this has occurred, it must be reduced by medication therapies or there must be an attempt to decrease the effect of the neoformation or of the perilesional brain edema on the rest of the nervous parenchyma by surgical decompression,
- to prevent the occurrence of internal hydrocephalus and, in the case of an already existing obstructive hydrocephalus, to decrease the volume of the ventricular CSF,
- to prevent endocranial circulatory disorders or to bring back to normal values the already affected cerebral sanguine circulation, in order to stop the development of the cerebral ischemia,
- in the case of certain signs that announce a complication, to stop the development of that particular process (decompression of the optic nerve in idiopathic ICH in order to stop the evolution of cecity, etc.),
- before the occurrence, or at the first signs of intracranial hypertension decompensation through the appearance of a cerebral hernia, to try various maneuvers for the protection of the nervous parenchyma by using methods such as ventricular drainage, sub-temporal decompressive craniectomy, craniectomy of posterior cerebral fosse with the excision of the posterior arch of the atlas, etc. [9,23,26,30,31,39,43]

Symptomatic Treatment

The symptomatic treatment is necessary in most cases of intracranial hypertension in order to decrease the intensity of the symptoms until the etiopathogenic therapy comes into effect, and then concomitantly with it. Antalgics, antiemetics, antivertigos, anticonvulsants, antithermics, sedatives, etc., are used, depending on the existing symptomatology. [1,2,21,43,47]

Therapeutic Schemes in Intracranial Hypertension

Treatment of the Brain Edema

The pathogenic treatment of the brain edema depends on the type of edema:

- the cellular cerebral (cytotoxic) edema occurs due to the intra/extracellular osmotic pressure disequilibrium, with an intact brain-blood barrier, and it is reduced by diuretics;
- the hydrostatic extracellular brain edema in hypertensive encephalopathy is caused by the increase in the hydrostatic pressure from the cerebral capillaries secondary to a severe AHT, and it is produced by an ultra-filtration mechanism with an intact brain-blood barrier;
- the oncotic (vasogenic) extracellular brain edema represents a severe alteration of the brain blood barrier (open brain-blood barrier), it has a peri-tumor development or in other lesions by through a vasogenic mechanism, and it responds favourably to corticosteroids;
- the mixed brain edema, cellular and extracellular, is the most frequent type of brain edema; the typical features occur from the start in the case of the traumatic brain edema.

Diuretics and corticosteroids are used in order to decrease the brain edema.[2,5,7,8,10]

The mannitol is an osmotic diuretic, and it is used in a dose of 0.25 – 1 g / Kgc intravenously; the effect occurs after 10 – 15 minutes, it lasts for approximately two hours and it may be repeated after 6 hours. It is efficient in the case of the brain edema with intact brain-blood barrier. The administration of larger doses does not reduce the intracranial pressure further, but there is a longer period of action. The mannitol must be carefully administered in order not to increase a hematoma by decreasing the volume of the parenchyma with an edema around. During the mannitol therapy, one must verify the serous osmolarity, which must be maintained between 300 – 315 mOsm / L.The osmolarity can be calculated, and must be maintained below 320 mOsm/ L.

The classical belief is that mannitol can be administered in sufficiently large doses, taking into account the serous osmolarity, in order to prevent a possible secondary renal insufficiency. Recent studies have specified the fact that the renal insufficiency, which can occur after the mannitol administration, is related more to the preexisting high blood pressureor to the existence of a diabetes mellitus, than to osmolarity or to the mannitol doses. [2,12,20,25,29]

Furosemide is an ansa diuretic, it is used in a dose of 10 – 40 mg, which is administered intravenously or as an initial dose of 0.5 – 1 mg / Kgc; it also decreases the CSF production.

The combination of these two diuretics is more efficient and it requires the monitoring of the sanguine electrolytes (potassium).

Corticosteroids (dexamethasone) are efficient in the vasogenic brain edema as they repair the brain-blood barrier. A quantity of 4 – 20 mg of dexamethasone is administered intravenously, and the effects are felt in a few hours. [12,33,36,52]

Decrease in CSF Secretion

Acetazolamide and corticosteroids reduce the production of cerebrospinal fluid, and they are used in order to reduce the CSF volume. Acetazolamide is a sulfonamide that specifically inhibits the carbonic anhydrase at the level of the renal tube, ciliary body, choroid plexus, and in the digestive mucous membrane. The acetazolamide administration in doses of 250 – 1000 mg / day gradually reduces the CSF production; it is necessary to monitor the electrolytes and the sanguine pH. [3,5,7,11,28,33]

A reduced CSF secretion also happens after the administration of mannitol and furosemide.

The rapid removal of the CSF excess can be performed by means of a ventricular drainage during the intracranial pressure monitoring, which ensures the intracranial pressure control, or by means of an external ventricular drainage in emergency cases. The CSF drainage by lumbar puncture or by lumbar catheter is not used due to the risk of cerebral herniation. In the case of an idiopathic intracranial hypertension syndrome, the lumbar-peritoneal shunt is sometimes used, while, in the case of an obstructive hydrocephalus, ventricular-peritoneal shunting systems may be used. [30,36,45,52]

Maintaining a Normal Cerebral Blood Perfusion

The sanguine arterial pressure increase is recommended in order to maintain an appropriate cerebral perfusion pressure when the monitoring reveals a significant increase in the intracranial pressure. The hypertensive therapy for the systemic blood pressure increase includes the administration of colloidal solutions, intravenous vasopressors, such as dopamine or phenylephrine. [1,8,10,15,26]

In the case of the intracranial hypertension syndrome in traumatic brain injury, the systemic blood pressure may usually increase up to 150 – 170 mm Hg. In the case of decreased values of the cerebral perfusion pressure, sanguine pressure increasing measures can be applied even with the risk of an ICP increase as the purpose is to maintain the normal values of the cerebral perfusion pressure. [32,35,46,49,50]

In the case of non-traumatic intracranial hypertension syndrome and in the absence of the cerebral hemorrhage, the blood pressure can increase up to 180 mm Hg.

Emergency Treatment Principles in Intracranial Hypertension

In the case of a patient with a suspicion of decompensating intracranial hypertension, one must perform and assess:

- the complete evaluation of the patient with the acute ICH syndrome: one must assess the consciousness level, the conscience state, the aspect of the pupils must be monitored and the Glasgow score must be established,
- the vital conditions: free aerial ways, respiration and the circulatory function; resuscitation operations are performed if needed, with oro-tracheal intubation, etc. In case of traumatisms, a cervical vertebral-medullar lesion must be excluded, and possible lesions with a vital risk must be revealed if they require an immediate solution.
- the emergency exploration by a cranial-cerebral computer tomography establishes the diagnosis and the therapeutic option is decided. [2,8,12,14,16,34]

Thus the first therapeutic actions are determined depending on the lesional characteristics:

- the expansive intracranial process (tumor, traumatic process), which has induced the ICH syndrome is surgically extirpated in order to remove the supplementary pathogenic volume with a compressive effect (mass effect), and which leads to a brain edema.
- the expansive intracranial process that blocks the CSF circulation paths with the production of an obstructive hydrocephalus and the ICH syndrome requires at first the performance of a ventricular drainage and then, based on the characteristics of the lesion, there will be an intervention for its extirpation.
- in the blood blockage of the ventricular system in intracranial hemorrhages, with the occurrence of the ICH syndrome due to obstructive hydrocephalus, the ventricular drainage is performed, and then the exploration and the treatment of the intracranial hemorrhage.
- the presence of a brain edema without any other lesion requires the anti-edematous treatment in order to reduce the intracranial pressure, at the same time as maintaining the a cerebral perfusion pressure within normal limits by the administration of mannitol, furosemide, dexamethasone, vasopressors, etc.
- in non-surgical multiple traumatic lesions, a pathogenic therapy is applied in order to decrease the intracranial pressure and stop the evolution of secondary traumatic lesions.
- an appropriate cerebral perfusion pressure must be maintained in order to prevent cerebral ischemia. PCP must be higher than 60 – 80 mm Hg.
- avoidance of the situations when the cerebral metabolism increases:

    - avoidance of stimuli: aspiration strictly when needed, patient's transportation,
    - hyperthermia must be vigorously discouraged: antithermic medication, muscular relaxing substances, cold packing up; the moderate hypothermia is an efficient procedure to decrease the cerebral metabolism and for cerebral protection.

- the evaluation of the biological parameters with the urgent control of the glycemia; in the case of the neurosurgical patient with a normal carbohydrate metabolism, it is not recommended to use glucose solutions as this may worsen the brain edema or the cerebral ischemic lesions

- the decrease in the arterial and intracranial venous blood volume by:
    - head raising, which facilitates the venous drainage and increases the CSF removal
    - the hyperventilation decreases PCO2 leading to an arterial vasoconstriction that decreases the cerebral sanguine volume
    - AT monitoring, in order to hinder AT variations: correction of the arterial hypotension (decrease in the cerebral sanguine perfusion), as well as of the high blood pressure(increase in the intracranial pressure)
    - pharmacologic methods to decrease the metabolism and the O2 needs with the reduction of the cerebral sanguine volume (thiopental 4-6 mg/kg or propofol 2-3 mg/kg), but with the cerebral perfusion pressure maintained within normal limits
    - the signs of ICH decompensation – unilateral mydriasis – (the cerebral compliance has been exceeded) require urgent measures of ICP decrease and in order to prevent a further ICP increase:
        - the occurrence of acute hydrocephalus (by any mechanism) imposes the CSF drainage with a ventricular catheter, which rapidly decreases the ICP
        - in order to prevent the cerebral herniation, a hemi-craniectomy can be used with a partial resection of the temporal lobe,
        - in cases of malign brain edema, which is resistant to medicine therapies, a hemi-craniectomy can be performed with the removal of the cranial bone and the sectioning of the dura mater in order to allow the expansion of the cerebral parenchyma during the acute stage,
        - in brainstem compressions, at the same time as the aggressive medication treatments, the decompression of the posterior cerebral fosse is performed by means of a sub-occipital craniectomy, completed by a ventricular drainage if there is also hydrocephalus.[34,37,40,42,50]

- in the case of an operated patient, with a post-surgery ICP monitoring, the normalization of the intracranial pressure values is monitored, as well as the improvement of the cerebral circulation:
    - if the cerebral perfusion pressure is below 70 mm Hg, the correction treatment of the intracranial blood contribution is started, even if the ICP is still high, by means of the administration of colloidal solutions, intravenous vasopressors, etc.
    - if the intracranial pressure has values of less than 20 mm Hg and the cerebral perfusion pressure is above 70 mm Hg, the patient is supervised, and the evolution of the ICP and PCP values are monitored.
    - if the intracranial pressure is higher than 20 mm Hg, the agitated patient is sedated and the permeability of the respiratory paths is checked; the head is raised at 25 - 30 degrees from horizontal, which leads to a moderate ICP decrease through an increase in the venous drainage. The ICP normalization during these

maneuvers does not require other therapeutic actions regarding the intracranial pressure.

- in the case of the patient who has not been in a surgery, but who has an ICP monitoring indication, one must survey and correct the intracranial pressure increases and the cerebral perfusion pressure decreases. The ICP values of more than 20 mm Hg require the agitated patient's sedation and the check of the respiratory path permeability. The decreased value of the cerebral perfusion pressure requires the specific therapy for the maintenance of the cerebral circulation within normal limits.

Treatment Scheme in Traumatic Acute Intracranial Hypertension

The therapeutic stages for patients with traumatic brain injury and an acute ICH syndrome aim to reduce the ICP increases and to maintain the PCP within normal limits. The treatment is performed progressively, depending on the monitoring values of ICP, PCP and of the other parameters. [2,7,8,12,14]

- sedation and perhaps a moderate hyperventilation; this is applied as long as ICP < 20 mm Hg for the first 12 hours:

- sedatives
- PaCO2 is maintained at ≈ 35 mm Hg in the case of mechanically ventilated patients
- when the ICP value is above 20 mm Hg, one must verify whether the increased pressure values are caused by the agitated state or if there is a mechanical obstruction that may cause the pressure increase. The patient who manifests a psycho-motor agitation is sedated, and, if ICP decreases below 20 mm Hg, the monitoring, as well as the pathogenic and symptomatic therapy in the intensive care ward are continued.

- CSF drainage with the ventricular catheter: if ICP > 20 mm Hg for more than 5 minutes, CSF drainage is used whenever needed, as long as the operation proves to be efficient.

- use of diuretics: if ICP is maintained high above 20 mm Hg for more than 5 minutes, the following procedures are used:

- osmotic diuresis: mannitol administration.
- loop diuretics: furosemide is used

The combination of these two diuretics is more efficient and is performed while monitoring of osmolarity and of the sanguine electrolytes.

- hyperventilation with the maintenance of PaCO2 at values of 25 – 30 mm Hg. Hyperventilation causes cerebral vasoconstriction and the ICP decrease by decreasing the cerebral sanguine flux. Hyperventilation is applied intermittently and it is recommended on the second day after a severe cranial-cerebral traumatism.

- hypertensive therapy for the increase in the systemic blood pressure, which can ensure a normal cerebral perfusion pressure if the intracranial pressure is increased. If cerebral contusion lesions are evident (areas of cerebral hemorrhage – hemorrhagic contusion), the systemic arterial pressure can increase up to 150 – 170 mm Hg; if there are no areas of cerebral contusion, the blood pressure can increase to 180 mm Hg.
- controlled hypothermia, maintaining an approximate temperature of 35 ° C.
- administration of a hypertonic NaCl solution with a concentration of 7.5 %.
- surgical decompression: if the cerebral CT exploration shows that the cerebral edema is very important without revealing a compressive intracranial lesion, performing a large decompressive craniectomy, unilateral or bilateral, must be considered.
- the anesthetic administration is performed with an electro-encephalic monitoring up to doses that diminish the EEG activity, using:

- non-barbituric hypnotic substances: etomidate, propofol.
- barbituric substances: phenobarbital, thiopental (barbituric coma).

- Trometamol administration (THAM), which generates a partial decrease in CO_2 pressure and produces a cerebral vasoconstriction. The condition is for the reactivity of the cerebral vessels to CO_2 to be intact
- the lumbar puncture of CSF drainage is applied after the exhaustion of the other therapeutic means. The cerebral computer tomography exploration must reveal the presence of the basal cisterns and of the lateral ventricles. The risk of inducing a cerebral hernia by this operation, which is not recommended in intracranial hypertension, is considered to be smaller than the unfavorable evolution by the accentuation of the intracranial pressure increase. [12,34,40,44,51]

Treatment Scheme in Intracranial Hypertension of Ischemic Stroke

The emergency treatment of the massive ischemic cerebral or cerebellar stroke, which may lead to an ICH syndrome, includes:

- securing the vital conditions: free aerial ways, respiration and circulatory function, in the circumstances of a critical condition or of a coma,
- the intravenous administration of a recombined activator of tissue plasminogen (rTPA, rtPA) during the first three hours from the beginning of the stroke in a dose of 0.9 mg/kg; maximum 90 mg. [1,13,17,18,24]

The intravenous administration of streptokinase or of other thrombolytic agents does not have the same effects as the rtPA administration.

- if it is necessary, a progressive decrease in the systemic blood pressure is performed,
- administration of osmotic diuretics (mannitol) if there are any signs of intracranial hypertension decompensation,
- hyperventilation when intracranial hypertension decompensation and cerebra hernia occurrence are imminent,

- cortico-therapy is not recommended in the treatment of the cerebral edema in cerebral ischemic stroke
- surgical intervention if the ICH decompensation occurs:

  - decompression and the evacuation of a cerebellar stroke with a compressive effect on the brainstem, perhaps a ventricular drainage too,
  - decompression and the evacuation of a massive cerebral hemispheric stroke, which can reduce the intracranial hypertension, but the surviving patients are left with major neurologic deficits. [27,32,34,35,38,41,47,48]

References

[1] Adams HP Jr, Brott TG, Crowell RM, et al. Guidelines for the management of patients with acute ischemic stroke: a statement for healthcare professionals from a special writing group of the Stroke Council, *American Heart Association. Circulation.* 1994; 90: 1588–1601.

[2] Adelson PD, Bratton SL, Carney NA, Chesnut RM, du Coudray HE,et al The use of barbiturates in the control of intracranial hypertension in severe pediatric traumatic brain injury. *Pediatr Crit Care Med.* 2003 ;4 :S49-52.

[3] Adelson PD, Bratton SL, Carney NA, Chesnut RM, et al The role of cerebrospinal fluid drainage in the treatment of severe pediatric traumatic brain injury. *Pediatr. Crit. Care Med.* 2003 , 4(3 Suppl):S38-9.

[4] Adelson PD, Bratton SL, Carney NA, Chesnut RM, et al Threshold for treatment of intracranial hypertension. *Pediatr. Crit. Care Med.* 2003 ;4(3 Suppl):S25-7.

[5] Adelson PD, Bratton SL, Carney NA, Chesnut RM, et al Use of hyperosmolar therapy in the management of severe pediatric traumatic brain injury. *Pediatr. Crit. Care Med.* 2003 ;4(3 Suppl):S40-4.

[6] Adelson PD, Bratton SL, Carney NA, Chesnut RM,et al Surgical treatment of pediatric intracranial hypertension. *Pediatr. Crit. Care Med.* 2003 ;4(3 Suppl):S56-9.

[7] Adelson PD, Bratton SL, Carney NA, Chesnut RM,et al The use of corticosteroids in the treatment of severe pediatric traumatic brain injury. *Pediatr. Crit. Care Med.* 2003 ;4(3 Suppl):S60-4.

[8] Adelson PD, Bratton SL, Carney NA,et al Critical pathway for the treatment of established intracranial hypertension in pediatric traumatic brain injury. *Pediatr. Crit. Care Med.* 2003 ;4(3 Suppl):S65-7.

[9] Allan R, Chaseling R. Subtemporal decompression for slit-ventricle syndrome: successful outcome after dramatic change in intracranial pressure wave morphology. Report of two cases. *J. Neurosurg.* 2004 ;101(Suppl):214-7.

[10] Battison C, Andrews PJ, Graham C, et al Randomized, controlled trial on the effect of a 20% mannitol solution and a 7.5% saline/6% dextran solution on increased intracranial pressure after brain injury. Crit. Care Med. 2005 ;33(1):196-202.

[11] Baxter P, Stack C, Short J. Treating head injuries. Studies of efficacy of medical and surgical interventions are urgently needed.*BMJ.* 2002 14;325(7377):1420.

[12] Berger S, Schwarz M, Huth R. Hypertonic saline solution and decompressive craniectomy for treatment of intracranial hypertension in pediatric severe traumatic brain injury. *J. Trauma.* 2002 53(3):558-63.

[13] Brandt T, von Kummer R, Muller-Kuppers M, Hacke W. Thrombolytic therapy of acute basilar artery occlusion: variables affecting recanalization and outcome. *Stroke.* 1996; 27: 875–881.

[14] Caricato A, Conti G, Della Corte F, Mancino A,et al Effects of PEEP on the intracranial system of patients with head injury and subarachnoid hemorrhage: the role of respiratory system compliance. *J. Trauma.* 2005 ;58(3):571-6.

[15] Coppage KH, Sibai BM. Treatment of hypertensive complications in pregnancy. *Curr. Pharm. Des.* 2005;11(6):749-57.

[16] Cruz J, Minoja G, Okuchi K. Major clinical and physiological benefits of early high doses of mannitol for intraparenchymal temporal lobe hemorrhages with abnormal pupillary widening: a randomized trial. *Neurosurgery.* 2002,;51(3):628-37.

[17] Demchuk AM, Burgin WS, Christou I, et al. Thrombolysis in brain ischemia (TIBI) transcranial Doppler flow grades predict clinical severity, early recovery, and mortality in patients treated with intravenous tissue plasminogen activator. *Stroke.* 2001; 32: 89–93.

[18] Diener HC, Ringelstein EB, von Kummer R, et al. Treatment of acute ischemic stroke with the low-molecular-weight heparin certoparin: results of the TOPAS trial: Therapy of Patients with Acute Stroke (TOPAS) Investigators. Stroke. 2001; 32: 22–29.

[19] Donnan GA, Davis SM. Surgical decompression for malignant middle cerebral artery infarction: a challenge to conventional thinking. *Stroke.* 2003 ;34(9):2307.

[20] Dziedzic T, Szczudlik A, Klimkowicz A, Rog TM, Slowik A. Is mannitol safe for patients with intracerebral hemorrhages? Renal considerations.*Clin. Neurol. Neurosurg.* 2003 ;105(2):87.

[21] Eckstein HH, Schumacher H, Dorfler A, et al. Carotid endarterectomy and intracranial thrombolysis: simultaneous and staged procedures in ischemic stroke. *J. Vasc. Surg.* 1999; 29: 459–471.

[22] El-Watidy S. Bifrontal decompressive craniotomy in a 6-month-old infant with posttraumatic refractory intracranial hypertension *Pediatr Neurosurg.*2005 ;41(3):151-4.

[23] Figaji AA, Fieggen AG, Peter JC. Early decompressive craniotomy in children with severe traumatic brain injury.*Childs Nerv. Syst.* 2003 ;19(9):666-73.

[24] Fraser JF, Hartl R. Decompressive craniectomy as a therapeutic option in the treatment of hemispheric stroke. *Curr .Atheroscler. Rep.* 2005 ;7(4):296-304.

[25] Georgiadis AL, Suarez JI. Hypertonic saline for cerebral edema. *Curr. Neurol. Neurosci. Rep.* 2003 ; 3(6):524-30

[26] Gupta R, Connolly ES, Mayer S, Elkind MS. Hemicraniectomy for massive middle cerebral artery territory infarction: a systematic review. *Stroke.* 2004 ;35(2):539-43

[27] Hacke W, Krieger D, Hirschberg M. General principles in the treatment of acute ischemic stroke. *Cerebrovasc. Dis.* 1991; 1 (suppl 1): 93–99.

[28] Iencean St M A new classification and a synergetical pattern in intracranial hypertension *Medical Hypotheses* , 2002 ;58(2):159-63.

[29] Iencean St M Brain edema - a new classification.*Medical Hypotheses* 2003;61(1):106-9.

[30] Jalan R. Pathophysiological basis of therapy of raised intracranial pressure in acute liver failure. *Neurochem Int.* 2005 ;47(1-2):78-83.

[31] Kamat P, Vats A, Gross M, Checchia PA. Use of hypertonic saline for the treatment of altered mental status associated with diabetic ketoacidosis. *Pediatr. Crit. Care Med.* 2003 ;4(2):239-42.

[32] Kasper GC, Wladis AR, Lohr JM, et al. Carotid thromboendarterectomy for recent total occlusion of the internal carotid artery. *J. Vasc. Surg.* 2001; 33: 242–250.

[33] Knapp JM. Hyperosmolar therapy in the treatment of severe head injury in children: mannitol and hypertonic saline.*AACN Clin Issues.* 2005 ;16(2):199-211.

[34] Kontopoulos V, Foroglou N, Patsalas J, et al Decompressive craniectomy for the management of patients with refractory hypertension: should it be reconsidered? *Acta Neurochir* (Wien).2002 ; 144(8):791-6.

[35] Kuo JR, Lin CL, Chio CC, Wang JJ, Lin MT. Effects of hypertonic (3%) saline in rats with circulatory shock and cerebral ischemia after heatstroke. *Intensive Care Med.*2003; 29(9):1567

[36] Lee AG, Pless M, Falardeau J,et al The use of acetazolamide in idiopathic intracranial hypertension during pregnancy. *Am. J. Ophthalmol.* 2005 ;139(5):855-9.

[37] Mathew P, Teasdale G, Bannan A, Oluoch-Olunya D. Neurosurgical management of cerebellar haematoma and infarct. J Neurol Neurosurg Psychiatry. 1995; 59: 287–292.

[38] McCormick PW, Spetzler RF, Bailes JE, Zabramski JM, Frey JL. Thromboendarterectomy of the symptomatic occluded internal carotid artery. *J. Neurosurg.* 1992; 76: 752–758.

[39] Owler BK, Parker G, Halmagyi GM, Pseudotumor cerebri syndrome: venous sinus obstruction and its treatment with stent placement. J. *Neurosurg.* 2003 ;98(5):1045-55.

[40] Schneider GH, Bardt T, Lanksch WR, Unterberg A. Decompressive craniectomy following traumatic brain injury: ICP, CPP and neurological outcome. *Acta Neurochir. Suppl.* 2002;81:77.

[41] Schwab S, Hacke W. Surgical decompression of patients with large middle cerebral artery infarcts is effective. *Stroke*. 2003 ;34(9):2304-5.

[42] Sebire G, Tabarki B, Saunders DE, Leroy I, et al Cerebral venous sinus thrombosis in children: risk factors, presentation, diagnosis and outcome. *Brain.* 2005 ;128(Pt 3):477-89.

[43] Serratrice J, Granel B, Conrath J,et al Benign intracranial hypertension and thyreostimulin suppression hormonotherapy.*Am. J. Ophthalmol.* 2002 ;134(6):910-1.

[44] Shiozaki T, Nakajima Y, Taneda M, etc all. Efficacy of moderate hypothermia in patients with severe head injury and intracranial hypertension refractory to mild hypothermia. *J. Neurosurg.* 2003 ;99(1):47-51.

[45] Tankisi A, Rolighed Larsen J, Rasmussen M, Dahl B, Cold GE. The effects of 10 degrees reverse trendelenburg position on ICP and CPP in prone positioned patients subjected to craniotomy for occipital or cerebellar tumours.*Acta Neurochir.* (Wien). 2002 ;144(7):665-70.

[46] Tisell M. How should primary aqueductal stenosis in adults be treated? A review.*Acta Neurol Scand.* 2005 ;111(3):145-53.

[47] Togay-Isikay C, Kim JY, Meads D, Tegeler C. Lumbar drainage affects transcranial Doppler pulsatility and waveforms in the presence of elevated intracranial pressure. *Eur. J. Neurol.* 2005 ;12(5):407-9.

[48] Treib J, Grauer MT, Woessner R, Morgenthaler M. Treatment of stroke on an intensive stroke unit: a novel concept. *Intensive Care Med.* 2000; 26: 1598–1611.

[49] Tsumoto T, Miyamoto T, Shimizu M, et al . Restenosis of the sigmoid sinus after stenting for treatment of intracranial venous hypertension: case report. *Neuroradiology* 2003; 45(12):911-5.

[50] Videtta W, Villarejo F, Cohen M, et al Effects of positive end-expiratory pressure on intracranial pressure and cerebral perfusion pressure. *Acta Neurochir. Suppl.* 2002;81:93-7.

[51] Vincent JL, Berre J. Primer on medical management of severe brain injury. *Crit. Care Med.* 2005 ;33(6):1392-9.

[52] Watling CJ, Cairncross JG. Acetazolamide therapy for symptomatic plateau waves in patients with brain tumors. Report of three cases. *J. Neurosurg.* 2002 ;97(1):224-6.

[53] Woodworth GF, McGirt MJ, Williams MA, Rigamonti D. The use of ventriculoperitoneal shunts for uncontrollable intracranial hypertension without ventriculomegally secondary to HIV-associated cryptococcal meningitis. *Surg. Neurol.* 2005 ;63(6):529-31;

Chapter XVI

Intracranial Hypotension

General Data

The intracranial hypotension represents the intracranial pressure decrease; theoretically, it may be generated by the decrease in the volume of any of the intracranial components: the cerebral parenchyma, the cerebrospinal fluid, and the sanguine content and/or by the rapid removal of a pathologic volume in the circumstances of a pressure equilibrium achieved by the efficient compensating mechanisms (especially in the case of chronic subdural hematomas).

The decrease in the volume of the cerebral parenchyma, by various mechanisms – senile cerebral atrophy, surgical resection, etc., does not generate first of all an intracranial hypotension syndrome, but there may be focal neurological symptoms depending on the cerebral areas that are suffering. The volume of the reduced cerebral parenchyma is progressively decreased by gliosis and/or by CSF; therefore, the intracranial pressure is maintained at normal values. The decrease in the intracranial sanguine volume by way of arterial hypotension leads to the decrease in the cerebral perfusion pressure with ischemic phenomena; this can also lead to a decreased CSF secretion, but the intracranial pressure decrease seems to be less important than ischemia. The surgical removal of a pathologic volume causes a sudden decrease in the endocranial volume and in the intracranial pressure, also known as the surgical cerebral-ventricular collapse, and which is rapidly compensated from a therapeutic point of view. Once the neurosurgical intervention has been performed, the endocranial cavity is no longer a closed environment, and there is no relationship between the intracranial hypotension and the surgical cerebral collapse. Therefore, of the three intracranial components, only the reduced volume of the cerebrospinal fluid intervenes in the occurrence of the intracranial hypotension. [4,8,15]

The intracranial hypotension is, therefore, the decrease in the intracranial pressure caused by the decrease in the volume of the cerebrospinal fluid secondary to the CSF loss. The intracranial hypotension is characterized by an orthostatic cephalea, exacerbated by coughing, laughing, the Valsalva maneuver, which is not calmed by antalgics and is accompanied by nausea, vomiting, vertigos, diplopia, etc. The diagnosis is confirmed by a lumbar manometry and by the paraclinical explorations performed (cisternography, CT scan, MRI).

From a clinical perspective, the intracranial hypotension can occur as:

- an acute form, with a violent symptomatology present in clinostatism, and which can evolve towards psychic disorders and changes in consciousness,
- a sub-acute form with absent symptoms or of a reduced intensity in clinostatism; they occur or they are exacerbated in orthostatism,
- a chronic, frequent form, with a symptomatology that occurs in orthostatism, with a lower, bearable intensity and a tiresome feeling that can allow undertaking an activity, though with a reduced efficiency. [16,21]

Etiology

The decrease in the normal CSF quantity in the cranial-spinal space can be caused by:

- the persistence of a dural continuity solution and the most frequent causes are the following ones:

- procedures involving the lumbar puncture: exploratory lumbar puncture, myelography, myelo-CT, rachianesthesia,
- cranial-spinal traumatisms with the generation of a CSF fistula,
- cranial-cerebral or spinal neurosurgical approaches,
- extremely rarely, by a spinal anterior-lateral CSF fistula in thoracic surgery,

- decrease in the CSF secretion by various mechanisms (after radiotherapy, etc.)
- reduced CSF quantity by a ventricular-peritoneal drainage,
- the so-called "spontaneous" intracranial hypotension, when none of the above-mentioned causes is evidenced, but the explorations prove the existence of several arachnoid fissures at the level of the spinal radicular sheath, or the case of the occult nasal CSF fistula.
- There have been cases of intracranial hypotension without the identification of a dural lesion in situations of dehydration, diabetic coma, uremia, or severe systemic illnesses.[4,8,17]

Pathogeny

There are two theories concerning the mechanism leading to the intracranial hypotension symptomatology:

- the decrease in the volume of cerebrospinal fluid leads to movements of the endocranial structures with traction of the formations that contain pain receptors: menunges, draining veins to sinuses, trigeminus, glossopharyngeal and vague nerves, as well as the first cervical spinal nerves. Orthostatism increases the traction of these structures, increasing the symptomatology.

- the decrease in the CSF volume leads to the intracranial pressure decrease and, therefore, according to the Monro–Kellie theory, a dilatation of the intracranial vascular structures occurs, which generates the accentuated cephalea in orthostatism. Moreover, there is a dilatation of the spinal epidural veins, explaining the spinal radicular pains.

It is currently thought that these two mechanisms are simultaneous, they act together and they explain the symptomatology. [9,12,13,22]

Clinical Presentation

The main symptom of the intracranial hypotension is the orthostatic cephalea: a cephalea that occurs or increases in orthostatism. The characteristics of the cephalea vary from one patient to another, but the common element is the fact that it is exacerbated in the orthostatic position, in a coughing effort, when laughing, etc., and it is not influenced by antalgics. [1,9,10,11,15]

Vertigo is the next symptom from the frequency point of view, vertigos occur or worsen in orthostatism too. There may also be feelings of nausea, vomiting, tingles, facial paresthesias, and radicular pains at the level of the superior limbs, all of which worsen in orthostatism.

Establishing the severity of the symptomatology and the etiology makes the distinction between the clinical forms: acute, sub-acute and chronic.

In the chronic form of intracranial hypotension, symptoms worsen in orthostatism, and they diminish or disappear in clinostatism. Sometimes, symptoms have a reduced intensity with the presence of an accentuated feeling of asthenia. Based on the dominating symptom, there are forms which are mainly cephalalgic, vertiginous, paresthesic, with vegetative disorders, etc.

In the sub-acute form, symptoms are manifested in the horizontal position, and they are exacerbated in orthostatism with an invalidating effect.

The acute form is characterized by an accentuated symptomatology, which is present in clinostatism, with vomiting, to dehydration, photophobia, sometimes even convulsive crises. Moreover, there may be psychic disorders or even modifications of the conscience state. The acute form is very rarely encountered nowadays. [17,18,20]

Paraclinical Explorations

The intracranial hypotension diagnosis implies the corroboration of the clinical data with the anamnesis, as well as the performance of certain explorations that may exclude other pathology and confirm the intracranial pressure decrease. In the context of certain maneuvers that include the lumbar puncture (myelography, myelo-CT, rachianesthesia), the occurrence of a clinical syndrome that announces the intracranial hypotension does not require the performance of other investigations in the case of a patient who has already undergone a cranial-cerebral exploration.

In the case of craniocerebral or spinal trauma, the investigations performed in order to establish the traumatic lesions show the dural lesion. [2,3,5,6]

The occurrence of the symptomatology at distance from a particular situation, which suggests the existence of a persistent dural fistula, requires the performance of certain explorations to establish the diagnosis. It is considered that the testing ~~of~~ a patient with chronic cephalea by arranging him or her in a Trendelenburg position, followed by the improvement of the cephalea, suggests a possible occult CSF fistula and it requires supplementary explorations.

The intracranial pressure measurement establishes the diagnosis, but it must be performed after the craniocerebral explorations that exclude another pathology. The cerebrospinal fluid has a quasi-normal composition; sometimes, there may be an increase in the cerebrospinal fluid proteins, lymphocytosis; erythrocytes can be present, with a xanthochromic aspect.

The craniocerebral computer tomography can prove the loss of the basal cisterns without the existence of a cerebral lesion.[5,719,22,24]

The cerebral MRI with a contrast substance can reveal:

- dura mater thickening,
- venous sinus dilatation,
- presence of certain subdural fluid collections,
- increase in the volume of the hypophysis gland,
- the movement of the brain downwards: the basal cisterns become smaller, there is an inferior motion of the optic chiasm, and sometimes the cerebellar amygdales descend.

The presence and intensity of these signs are in direct relation to the clinical gravity, and the improvement of the symptomatology is accompanied by the attenuation and erasure of the MNR modifications.

The radioactive isotope cisternography shows the CSF fistulas:

- directly, by noticing the radio-isotopic accumulation outside the sub-arachnoid space, or
- indirectly, by not outlining the radio-isotope at the level of the cerebral convexity and the notification of the latter in urine or in the adipose tissue.

The computer myelography (myelo-CT) shows the CSF spinal fistulas right at the level of the cranium base.

Treatment

The intracranial hypotension treatment is:

- etiologic, and it consists of closing the CSF fistula,
- pathogenic, which consists of recreating the normal CSF volume, and
- symptomatic, which refers to the treatment of the symptoms related to intracranial hypotension.

As the intracranial hypotension syndrome frequently occurs after the lumber puncture, the pathogenic and symptomatic treatment is often in the foreground, waiting for the dural orifice produced by the lumbar puncture to become obstruent.

The symptomatic treatment of cephalea consists in avoiding the orthostatism, having the patient rest in bed, and the oral or intravenous administration of caffeine or theophyline. Xanthins (theophyline) also increase the vascular resistance in the cerebral territory, reducing the circulation and diminishing the venous dilatation. Bed rest decreases the CSF pressure in the spinal dural sac and at the level of the remaining lumbar puncture orifice.

The CSF volume is recovered by oral and intravenous hydration, as well as by the administration of mineral corticoids.

Depending on the development, it can be ascertained whether the dural orifice of the lumbar puncture is maintained and if the CSF loss persists. In this case, a "patch" applying operation is performed at the level of the dural puncture orifice. The epidural blood patch is achieved by an autologous blood injection in the epidural space at the level of the previously performed lumbar puncture, with very good results; this operation needs to be repeated only very rarely.

The surgical solution of the CSF fistula is applied from the very beginning in traumatic dural lesions (cranial-cerebral wound, vertebral-medullar wound, cranium base fracture with CSF fistula, etc.), or the surgery may be temporized based on the intensity of the CSF loss and on the fistula location, with therapeutic protection, supervising its spontaneous closure (in the CSF fistula from the cranium base fracture). There may also be surgical solutions for the spinal dural lesions remaining after the lumbar puncture only if none of the previously presented procedures has proven to be efficient. [12,14,16]

References

[1] Albayram S, Wasserman BA, Yousem DM, et al: Intracranial hypotension as a cause of radiculopathy from cervical epidural venous engorgement: case report. *AJNR* 23:618–621, 2002

[2] Alvarez-Linera J, Escribano J, Benito-Leon J, et al: Pituitary enlargement in patients with intracranial hypotension syndrome. *Neurology* 55:1895–1897, 2000

[3] Benamor M, Tainturier C, Graveleau P, et al: Radionuclide cisternography in spontaneous intracranial hypotension. *Clin. Nucl. Med* 23:150–151, 1998

[4] Binder DK, Sarkissian V, Dillon WP, Weinstein PR. Spontaneous intracranial hypotension associated with transdural thoracic osteophyte reversed by primary dural repair. Case report. *J. Neurosurg Spine.* 2005 ;2(5):614-8.

[5] Brightbill TC, Goodwin RS, Ford RG: Magnetic resonance imaging of intracranial hypotension syndrome with pathophysiological correlation. *Headache* , 2000, 40:292–299

[6] Bruera O, Bonamico L, Giglio JA, et al: Intracranial hypotension: the nonspecific nature of MRI findings. *Headache* , 2000, 40: 848–852

[7] Chen CC, Luo CL, Wang SJ, et al: Colour Doppler imaging for diagnosis of intracranial hypotension. *Lancet*,1999, 354:826–829

[8] Davenport RJ, Chataway SJ, Warlow CP: Spontaneous intracranial hypotension from a CSF leak in a patient with Marfan's syndrome. *J. Neurol. Neurosurg Psychiatry*,1995, 59:516–519

[9] Dickerman RD, Morgan J. Pathogenesis of subdural hematoma in healthy athletes: postexertional intracranial hypotension? Acta Neurochir (Wien). 2005;147(3):349-50

[10] Evan RW, Mokri B: Spontaneous intracranial hypotension resulting in coma. *Headache*,2002, 42:159–160

[11] Ferrante E, Savino A. Thunderclap headache caused by spontaneous intracranial hypotension. *Neurol .Sci.* 2005 ;26 Suppl 2

[12] Fishman RA, Dillon WP: Dural enhancement and cerebral displacement secondary to intracranial hypotension. *Neurology*,1993, 43:609–611

[13] Good DC, Ghobrial M: Pathologic changes associated with intracranial hypotension and meningeal enhancement on MRI. *Neurology,*1993, 43:2698–2700

[14] Hannerz J, Dahlgren G, Irestedt L, Meyerson B, Ericson K. Treatment of idiopathic intracranial hypotension: cervicothoracic and lumbar blood patch and peroral steroid treatment. *Headache.* 2006 Mar;46(3):508-11

[15] Hong M, Shah GV, Adams KM, et al: Spontaneous intracranial hypotension causing reversible frontotemporal dementia. *Neurology* ,2002,58:1285–1287

[16] Iencean St M A new classification and a synergetical pattern in intracranial hypertension. *Medical Hypotheses* , 2002 ;58(2):159-63.

[17] Inenaga C, Tanaka T, Sakai N, et al: Diagnostic and surgical strategies for intractable spontaneous intracranial hypotension. Case report. *J. Neurosurg,*2001, 94:642–645

[18] Kong DS, Park K, Nam do H, Lee JI, Kim JS, Eoh W, Kim JH. Clinical features and long-term results of spontaneous intracranial hypotension. *Neurosurgery.* 2005 57(1):91-6

[19] Koss SA, Ulmer JL, Hacein-Bey L: Angiographic features of spontaneous intracranial hypotension. *AJNR* ,2003, 24:704–706

[20] Kremer S, Taillandier L, Schmitt E, Bologna S, Moret C, Picard L, Bracard S. Atypical clinical presentation of intracranial hypotension: coma. *J.Neurol* 2005; 252 (11):1399-400

[21] Moriyama E, Nishida A. Intracranial hypotension.*J. Neurosurg.* 2005;102(5):964-5.

[22] Schievink WI, Akopov SE. Filum ependymoma mimicking spontaneous intracranial hypotension. *Headache.* 2005 ;45(5):607-9.

[23] Schievink WI, Maya MM, Tourje J, Moser FG. Pseudo-subarachnoid hemorrhage: a CT-finding in spontaneous intracranial hypotension. *Neurology.* 2005,12;65(1):135-7.

[24] Takahashi M, Momose T, Kameyama M, Mizuno S, Kumakura Y, Ohtomo K. Detection of cerebrospinal fluid leakage in intracranial hypotension with radionuclide cisternography and blood activity monitoring. *Ann. Nucl. Med.* 2005;19(4):339-43.

Addendum

Pressure measure units

1 Pa = 1 N / 1 m^2 = (1 Kg m / sec^2) / 1 m^2

1 atm = 1.01325 • 10^5 Pa

1 bar = 1 • 10^5 Pa

1 Torr = 1 mm Hg = 1.3332 • 10^2 Pa = 133,3 Pa

1 atm = 760 Torr = 760 mm Hg

1 KPa = 7.5 mm Hg = 102 mm H_2O = 10.2 cm H_2O

1 mm Hg = 13.6 mm H_2O

1 cm H_2O = 0.735 mm Hg, 10 cm H_2O = 7.35 mm Hg

Index

A

B

C

D

E

F

G

H

I

J

K

L

M

N

O

P

T

U

V

W

X

Y